Monitoring Positive Pressure Therapy in Sleep-Related Breathing Disorders

Vivien Schmeling Piccin

Monitoring Positive Pressure Therapy in Sleep-Related Breathing Disorders

Advanced Analysis of Respiratory Flow Curves

Springer

Vivien Schmeling Piccin
Sao Paulo, SP, Brazil

ISBN 978-3-031-50291-0 ISBN 978-3-031-50292-7 (eBook)
https://doi.org/10.1007/978-3-031-50292-7

This Springer imprint is published by the registered company Springer Nature Switzerland AG
The registered company address is: Gewerbestrasse 11, 6330 Cham, Switzerland

Paper in this product is recyclable

For Roberto, Priscila, and Andressa

Foreword

Providing good sleep quality for people with sleep-related breathing disorders is a significant challenge for respiratory physiotherapists and other professionals working in the field. These patients chronically suffer from the negative effects of interrupted sleep, constant hypoxia, increased respiratory effort, and disturbing arousal. Some of them are strongly symptomatic, others not so much. Regardless of the presence or lack of symptoms, we must always prioritize the comfort and effectiveness of positive pressure treatment. Contrary to what many people think, the adherence program to positive pressure devices in the sleeping field goes far beyond simply programming a device and choosing a mask.

Even with all our willingness as a professional, if knowledge about technology, access to information, and quality training are not constant, our role as a facilitator in the process of adapting to positive pressure devices will be flawed. This point is critical! Without training and constant actualization, we end up inadvertently contributing to the patient giving up on positive pressure therapy, and their treatment discontinuation is most likely due to our fault.

Analyzing respiratory flow curves and knowing how to interpret them enriches, clarifies, and complements the objective of assessing treatment-related complaints. Going deeper into the understanding of this resource increases the chances of treatment success and improves problem-solving, favoring patient’s therapy adherence and the positive results that come from it.

Vivien Schmeling Piccin's work provides the reader with a complete, comprehensive, and didactic approach to the advanced analysis of the patient's respiratory flow curves during sleeping, reflecting the author's years of study and clinical practice. Now it's all about enjoying the book!

Flávia Baggio Nerbass

Sleep Laboratory/Heart Institute (InCor)
University of Sao Paulo Medical School/FMUSP
Sao Paulo, SP, Brazil

Heart Institute (InCor)/FMUSP
Sao Paulo, SP, Brazil

Brazilian Association of Cardiorespiratory
Physiotherapy and Physiotherapy in Intensive Care
(ASSOBRAFIR)
Sao Paulo, SP, Brazil

Preface

What is the importance of assessing respiratory flow curves during sleep? I have so many answers to this question that I am concerned about not being able to put the magnitude of its importance into words. First, I think that everyone is unique, and just like fingerprints, I believe that sleep breathing patterns give unique characteristics to each person. Understanding how a person is breathing when using a pressure device to treat sleep breathing disorders is a piece of precious information to properly conduct the treatment (especially in the most challenging cases). By analyzing the respiratory flow curve, we can verify if the therapeutic pressure is adequate, if we are not committing iatrogeny (through sub-therapeutic or excessive pressure), and understand the patient's phenotypic pattern (high or low loop gain). We can also verify the existence of associated comorbidities (for example, chronic obstructive pulmonary disease, congestive heart failure) and observe any pathological breathing pattern that may have been triggered by body fluid displacement during the night. We can even, in an allusion to the famous detective Sherlock Holmes (the fictional British literature character created by Sir Arthur Conan Doyle), investigate, using the respiratory flow curve data, if sleep distribution is adequate, if sleep architecture is recovered, whether the patient is taking the medications correctly, and if the health team is positioning the patient in the proper position while sleeping! The possibilities are endless, and the reader will discover this throughout the course of the book.

Of course, I cannot deny the merit of a good anamnesis, the direct conversation with the patient, and the importance of the remote monitoring system that helps us so much in patient follow-up. Everything is important and irreplaceable! But the respiratory flow curve analysis adds to all this. It is a powerful tool for patient follow-up, and once we know its possibilities, we will never leave it aside. However, for great use of this tool, we also need a good basic knowledge of physiology and pathophysiology of sleep and the respiratory system. Understanding the breathing pattern in the different stages of sleep, knowing underlying diseases that can influence respiratory dynamics, the normal morphology of the respiratory flow curve, and possible causes for the alteration of this normality, among other topics, are fundamental, as everything is interconnected. Therefore, in this book, I address some of these subjects, without intending to educate anyone, but remember the importance of this knowledge for an adequate interpretation of the respiratory flow curves.

Thus, this book aims not only to present the analysis of the respiratory flow curves during sleep and the importance of this but also to help the reader understand the influence of the physiological and pathophysiological processes on the respiratory flow curve pattern during sleep. Only with this understanding and making the best use of the instruments we have (the respiratory flow curve analysis included!), we will be able to correctly apply the precision medicine concept, in its broad sense.

I hope you enjoy the book and that the reading can be a transformative experience!

Sao Paulo, SP, Brazil Vivien Schmeling Piccin

Acknowledgments

Cláudia Albertini, my journey with sleep began because of you! So, my first acknowledgment goes to you. Thank you for being such a wonderful friend in my life!

Then, "Gegê" welcomed me to the Sleep Laboratory at Instituto do Coração and it was there that I consolidated my knowledge base on sleep. You are a person I admire a lot. A true master and a special human being. I will never forget the hug you gave me when I lost my mother. Thank you Dr. Geraldo Lorenzi-Filho!

I would like to say a huge thank you to my dear friend Rafaela Andrade who kindly took the time to review this book. Rafaela has been a great partner for me in projects and in life. God has blessed me with marvelous people around me and she is certainly one of them!

Many thanks to my friend Flavia Nerbass for her support. My work of disseminating knowledge about the importance of analyzing respiratory flow curves began more than ten years ago, and I could always count on Flavia's support in this matter.

I've made many friends along the way and I am afraid that if I make a list, someone will get left off, and that wouldn't be fair. So, thanks to all my friends in the sleep field and from different backgrounds in the health area. You were all crucial to my academic and personal training!

More than anything I would like to thank all the patients with whom I've had contact, directly or indirectly. My sincere thanks for teaching me so much!

Contents

Abbreviations and Acronyms

AASM	American Academy of Sleep Medicine
AC	Alternating current
CSA	Central sleep apnea
TECSA	Treatment-emergent central sleep apnea
OSA	Obstructive sleep apnea
AutoSet™	Trade name for ResMed's algorithm for automated continuous positive airway pressure equipment
cmH_2O	Centimeters of water
CO_2	Carbon dioxide
CPAP	Continuous positive airway pressure
DC	Direct current
SRBD	Sleep-related breathing disorder
EPAP	Expiratory positive airway pressure
$EtCO_2$	End-tidal of carbon dioxide
HR	Heart rate
Hz	Hertz
AHI	Apnea-hypopnea index
ICSD	International Classification of Sleep Disorders
IPAP	Inspiratory positive airway pressure
L/min	Liters per minute
LG	Loop gain
lpm	Liters per minute
NREM	Non-rapid eye movement
O_2	Oxygen
PAP	Positive airway pressure
$PaCO_2$	Partial pressure of carbon dioxide in arterial blood
PaO_2	Partial pressure of oxygen in arterial blood
REM	Rapid eye movement
RERA	Respiratory effort-related arousals
ResScan™	Trade name for ResMed´s data management software for positive pressure equipment

SaO_2	Oxygen saturation
Sec	Second
OHS	Obesity hypoventilation syndrome
SmartStart™	Trade name for ResMed's system for automatic CPAP activation and deactivation (automatically turns on the device when the patient breathes through the mask and automatically turns off the equipment when the patient removes the mask)
UARS	Upper airway resistance syndrome (also known as RERA: respiratory effort-related arousal)
UA	Upper airway

Part 1
Monitoring Positive Pressure Therapy in Sleep-Related Breathing Disorders: Advanced Analysis of Respiratory Flow Curves/Fundamentals

In this section of the book, we present normal sleep and sleep-disordered breathing and aspects of the treatment and monitoring of positive airway pressure. We present respiratory flow curves (how to analyze these curves) and important aspects of positive airway pressure device algorithms, used for the treatment of sleep-disordered breathing. Also provided in this section are examples of flow curves and other advanced graphics.

Chapter 1
Sleep

1.1 Sleep and Its Characteristics

Humans exhibit circadian rhythms of approximately 24 h that are self-sustaining in physiology and behavior, which are regulated by a central clock in the hypothalamus [1]. This system plays a role in the regulation of diverse physiological functions such as central body temperature, hormone release, and sleep. The sleep-wake cycle is the most evident circadian rhythm in men and women, and its main stimulus is ambient light.

When we sleep, there is a change in our state of consciousness and we restore our balance, preserving various functions such as immunity, metabolism, cognition, cardiovascular activity, and humor, among many others. Several studies have already shown that poor sleep quality increases the risk of disorders in the body (e.g., increased blood pressure, cardiovascular diseases, diabetes, and depression) [2, 3].

Nowadays we know that sleeping well is essential for our physical and mental health. Unfortunately, modern lifestyles often lack regular working, eating, and sleeping patterns. And despite reports on the occurrence of sleep disorders dating back to ancient times, this field of medicine has only recently received greater attention [4, 5].

Sleep is physiological, necessary, temporary, reversible, and cyclical [6]. It is an active process, with variation and duration controlled by specific structures in the central nervous system, and can be divided into two distinct states: REM (rapid eye movement) and NREM (non-rapid eye movement). REM sleep only has one stage, while NREM has three different sleep stages called N1, N2, and N3 (in an increasing degree of depth of sleep, respectively) [4, 5].

The sleep set in which all stages of NREM (N1, N2, and N3) and REM sleep are completed is called a sleep cycle and in a normal individual, the sleep cycle lasts between 70 and 110 min, repeating 4–6 times throughout the night (Fig. 1.1) [4].

V. S. Piccin, *Monitoring Positive Pressure Therapy in Sleep-Related Breathing Disorders*, https://doi.org/10.1007/978-3-031-50292-7_1

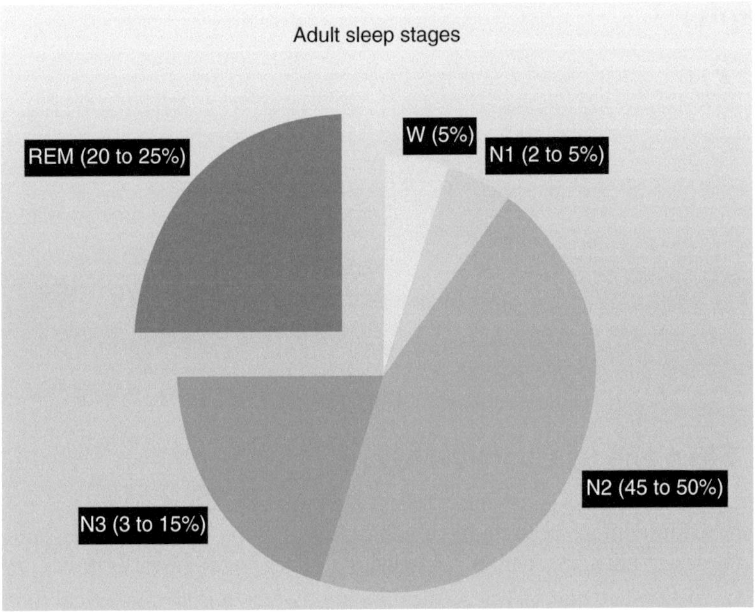

Fig. 1.1 Percentage classification of the various sleep stages in adults. Wake (W) in sleep represents less than 5% of the night. The N1 stage generally accounts for 2–5% of sleep; N2 for 45–50% of sleep; and the N3 stage for 3–15% of sleep (NREM sleep is usually 75–80% of sleep). REM (rapid eye movement) sleep generally accounts for 20–25% of sleep time [7]. (Figure source: own work)

NREM and REM sleep have different characteristics regarding endocrine, respiratory, cardiovascular, gastrointestinal, and genitourinary functions. Mainly, in NREM sleep we observe regular ventilation, maintenance of effectiveness of the proprioceptive and chemoreceptive reflexes, active intercostal muscles, maintenance of upper airway muscle tone, eurhythmic decrease in heart rate, and a regular decrease in blood pressure and cardiac output. In REM sleep there is a varied range of ventilation, the proprioceptive and chemoreceptor reflexes are canceled, intercostal muscles become inactive, muscle tone in the upper airways is reduced, heart rate becomes variable, and blood pressure and cardiac output fluctuate irregularly. REM sleep is also known as paradoxical sleep just because of the paradox of being a period when our mind is more active and muscle tone is more relaxed [4, 8]. Figure 1.2 shows the relationship between human sleep, level of consciousness patterns, and electroencephalogram (EEG).

The distribution of sleep stages during the night can be altered by several factors such as age, circadian rhythm, room temperature, drug ingestion, or by certain diseases. But normally, NREM sleep is more concentrated in the first part of the night, while REM sleep predominates in the second part [4, 8].

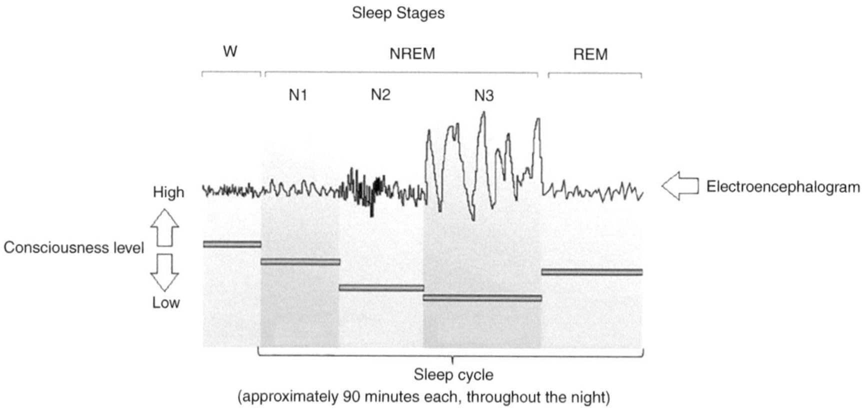

Fig. 1.2 Sleep stages are characterized by differences in the frequency and amplitude of the electroencephalographic (EEG) waves. Stage N1 includes light sleep with low-amplitude waveforms. Stage N2 is characterized by sleep spindles (high-frequency waves) and K complexes (not shown). Stage N3 represents slow wave sleep (SWS), with high amplitude waves and a deeper level of unconsciousness. These three stages comprise non-rapid eye movement (NREM) sleep. The subsequent stage is rapid eye movement (REM) sleep, which is associated with a higher level of consciousness. (Modified after Bryant et al., 2004 (with permission) [8])

1.2 Respiration While Sleeping

Recalling respiratory physiology, we know that the main function of our lungs is to exchange O2 and CO2 between blood and gas and thus maintain normal levels of PaO_2 and $PaCO_2$ in arterial blood. PaO_2 and $PaCO_2$ values remain at adequate levels mainly because ventilation is carefully maintained by our organism [9]. This regulation of gas exchange is sustained by three basic elements of the respiratory control system: (1) the sensors, which capture the information of circulating blood gas levels and, afferently, feed the (2) central controller in the brain, which coordinates the information and sends impulses to the (3) effectors (respiratory muscles), which promote ventilation. By means of a complex neural network, the respiratory muscles in the chest wall perform their function [9]. Figure 1.3 shows these basic elements of the respiratory control system [10].

The most important factor to control ventilation under normal conditions is $PaCO_2$, which can be very sensitive to minor changes. For example, a reduction in $PaCO_2$ may reduce ventilation, and even generate a central apnea or hypopnea event, in an attempt to re-establish normal values of $PaCO_2$ in arterial blood (between 35 and 45 mmHg), as shown in Fig. 1.4 [12].

The intensity of the body's response to $PaCO_2$ changes also depends on another factor, called cyclical neuroanatomic interaction or loop gain. The stability of the respiratory system is dictated by the magnitude of the loop gain. If the magnitude of the ventilatory response is high (hyperpnea) about the magnitude of the disorder (hypopnea), in other words, a high gain loop, ventilation will be unstable and will fluctuate between hyperpnea and hypopnea/apnea. In contrast, if the magnitude of

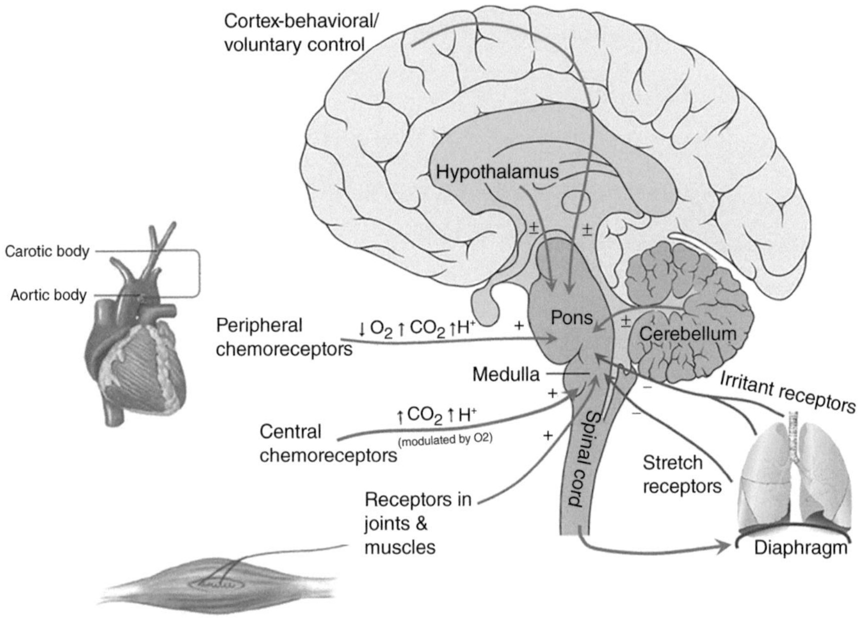

Fig. 1.3 The basic elements of respiratory control: sensors (central and peripheral chemoreceptors, receptors in the lung, and other receptors), which capture information and feed the central controller; the central controller in the brain (bridge, spinal cord, and other parts of the brain), which coordinates information and sends impulses to effectors; and effectors (respiratory muscles) promote ventilation. (Modified after Carroll, 2010 (with permission) [11])

the response is low, i.e., a low loop gain, the ventilation will remain stable in response to the disturbance. That is to say, the breathing pattern is the result of a balance between "Control Gain" (represented by the sensitivity of central and peripheral chemoreceptors to CO_2 variations) and "Plain Gain" (represented by the effectiveness of the lungs in altering blood gases and the ability to anatomically support the upper airway, especially during the various sleep phases) (Fig. 1.5) [13].

Typically, we observe that there is a high loop gain in the occurrence of central apnea/hypopnea at the beginning of pressure therapy to treat sleep apnea. This usually occurs because individuals with obstructive sleep apnea (particularly severe) often have higher values of $PaCO_2$ in their blood, even if they are in the normal $PaCO_2$ range. When these people begin to treat apnea with a positive pressure device, the $PaCO_2$ values decrease due to the support of the upper respiratory tract through the pneumatic effect of positive pressure, which normalizes ventilation.

However, the breathing control center, in the central nervous system, may not be equalized to work with the new $PaCO_2$ values, and can respond with central apneas/hypopneas in an attempt to return the usual $PaCO_2$ rates [13]. Likewise, depending on the loop gain (sensitivity) of each individual, the initial stimulus (in this example, central apnea) can generate an increased response (hyperventilation), leading to treatment-emergent central sleep apnea (Fig. 1.6) [13–16].

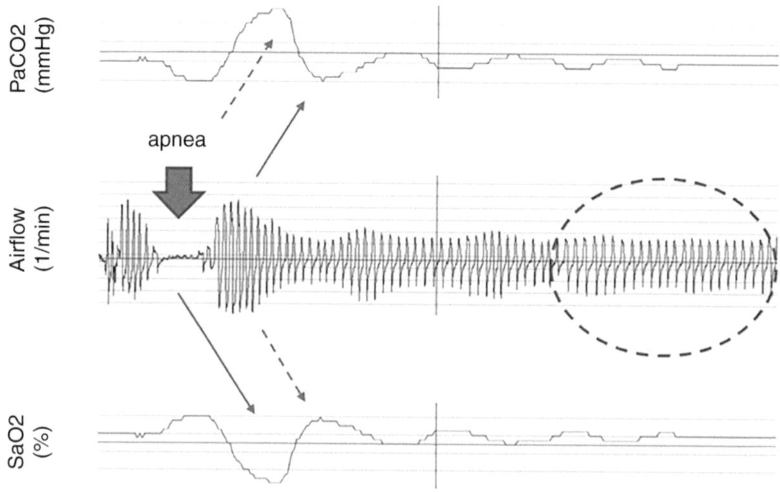

Fig. 1.4 Ventilatory response to carbon dioxide changes. In this example, we can see that, from an apnea event, there is an increase (dotted line) in CO_2 and a reduction in SaO_2 (straight line). The hyperventilation response after the apnea event generates a decrease in CO_2 level (straight line) and an increase in SaO_2 (dotted line). The difference between the accumulation of CO_2 during respiratory disorders (hypopnea or apnea) and the elimination of CO_2 during the subsequent intervening period determines the CO_2 balance and the breathing pattern normalization during sleep (highlighted by the dotted circle). (Source: own work)

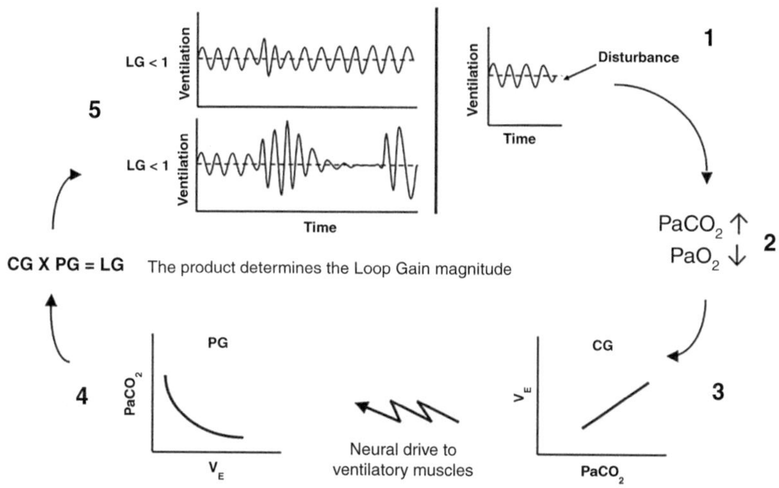

Fig. 1.5 When a ventilatory disorder (1) occurs (e.g., sleep apnea or hyperventilation event), the result is a variation in CO_2, to a greater or lesser extent (2). This variation must be detected by the central and peripheral chemoreceptors (3) ("Control Gain"), and the sensitivity of these sensors will influence the neural response/stimulus sent to the ventilatory muscles. The effectiveness of the lungs and upper airway (4) ("Plain Gain") will also influence the balance of the gain loop (the magnitude of the response). Thus, the product of "Control Gain" versus "Plain Gain" will be the ventilatory response, which may be exacerbated (high loop gain>1) or not (low loop gain <1) (5). (Modified after Deacon-Diaz, 2018 (with permission) [13])

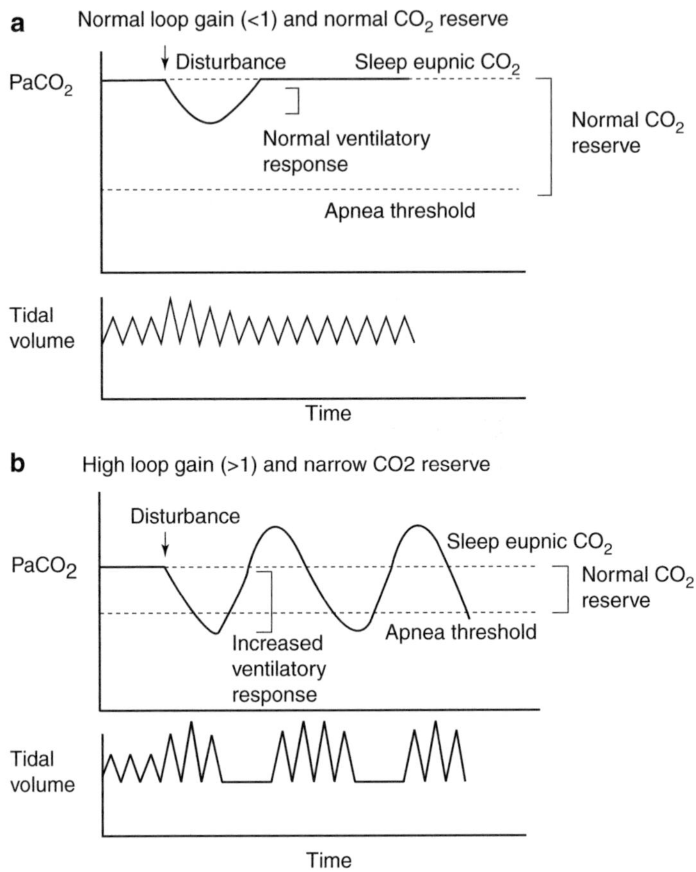

Fig. 1.6 Loop gain (LG) in central apnea during sleep. In panel a, a subject with ventilatory stability demonstrates an appropriate ventilatory response (normal loop gain, or LG < 1) to a disturbance. In panel b, a subject with ventilatory instability manifests an increased ventilatory response (high loop gain, or LG > 1) resulting in a cycle of hyperventilation and central apneas. Black arrow = disturbance causing hyperventilation (e.g., arousal, hypercapnia, hypoxia). (Source: Hernandez & Patil, 2016 (with permission))

In respiratory flow curve analysis when using positive pressure equipment, we will often encounter events related to CO_2 variations during sleep determined by the inherent response of each organism (loop gain) to respiratory events.

1.3 Respiratory Sleep Disorders

During normal sleep, respiratory system functions are maintained (oxygen supply, removal of carbon dioxide, and maintenance of the acid-base balance). The respiratory center is in the medulla oblongata and pons (in the brainstem), and correctly modulates the respiratory system. It is responsible for generating and maintaining the respiratory rhythm, and for adjusting it in homeostatic response to physiological changes. The respiratory center receives input from chemoreceptors, mechanoreceptors, the cerebral cortex, and the hypothalamus to regulate the rate and depth of breathing. This center is stimulated by altered levels of oxygen, carbon dioxide, and blood pH, by stress- and anxiety-related hormonal changes from the hypothalamus, and by signals from the cerebral cortex to give conscious control of breathing [5, 12, 17].

However, due to the specific characteristics of the functioning of our organism in NREM and REM sleep, associated with factors such as obesity, aging, and craniofacial changes, among others, sleep is associated with many derangements [5, 12, 17]. The International Classification of Sleep Disorders (ICSD) [18] helps provide a standardized classification and definitions for sleep disorders. Specifically, the third edition of the ICSD (ICSD-3) includes insomnia, central disorders of hypersomnolence, sleep-wake circadian rhythm disorders, parasomnia, sleep-related movement disorders, and sleep-related breathing disorders.

The causes of sleep-related breathing disorders (SRBD) range from breathing control of upper airway and chest wall mechanics, causing compromised ventilatory and resistive loading [19]. SRBD include obstructive sleep apnea (OSA), central sleep apnea (CSA), hypoventilation, and upper airway resistance syndrome (UARS, also known as RERA: Respiratory Effort-Related Arousals).

Sleep-related breathing disorders (SRBD) refer to abnormal breathing patterns or an abnormal gas exchange reduction that occurs during sleep. They mainly include obstructive sleep apnea (OSA), central sleep apnea (CSA), hypoventilation, and upper airway resistance syndrome (UARS, also known as RERA: Respiratory Effort-Related Arousals). During sleep, but usually associated with the use of positive pressure therapy, another breathing disorder that can be observed is treatment-emergent central sleep apnea (TECSA), previously described in the literature as complex apnea [12, 20].

In OSA, upper airway patency is compromised by a combination of several factors including anatomy, and muscle activity, among others. OSA is the most frequent respiratory sleep disorder and is characterized by repetitive episodes of complete or partial obstruction of the upper airways during sleep (obstructive apnea or hypopnea, respectively), followed by drops in oxyhemoglobin saturation and/or arousals [14].

In a CSA, respiratory flow is absent, due to a lack of respiratory effort (could be a physiological manifestation of different processes such as high altitude, narcotics, and cardiovascular disease, among others). During a central apnea event, there may also be reduced activity of the pharyngeal dilator muscles. This reduction associated with the absence of airflow can lead to the upper airway patency collapse after the beginning of a central respiratory event. This phenomenon is classified as mixed apnea [14, 21].

TECSA is a well-known phenomenon characterized by the development or persistence of central apneas or hypopneas during the application of continuous positive airway pressure (but may also occur with almost all alternative treatments for OSA management and not only with PAP-therapies) [22]. In general, these patients have predominantly obstructive apneas during the diagnostic sleep study, and no clinical characteristics that can distinguish patients who develop TECSA from patients with normal response to sleep apnea treatment. This pattern likely occurs due to an exacerbated response of the respiratory center to stimuli coming from the chemoreceptors (mostly because of $PaCO_2$ changes), at the start of treating obstructive sleep apnea with positive pressure equipment (high loop gain, and we will talk more about this topic later). In a broader perspective, any occurrence of significant central apnea activity during attempts to restore airway permeability with positive pressure equipment can be classified as TECSA [23–25].

Hypoventilation occurs when ventilation is insufficient to meet metabolic needs at the alveolar level. It is characterized by an increase in the partial pressure of carbon dioxide ($PaCO_2$) in arterial blood. The ability to maintain an adequate level of ventilation depends on three factors: integrity of the respiratory muscles, the workload to which the respiratory muscles are subjected, and adequacy of the central nervous system command to breathe. The imbalance of one or more of these factors leads to the risk of hypoventilation. Hypoventilation can be related to neuromuscular disorders (such as, e.g., Duchenne muscular dystrophy), disorders of the central nervous system (such as congenital central hypoventilation syndrome), thoracic deformities (such as, e.g., severe scoliosis), and obesity. Obesity hypoventilation syndrome (OHS) is defined by the presence of daytime alveolar hypoventilation ($PaCO_2$>45 mmHg) among patients with a body mass index ≥30 kg/m^2, in the absence of other causes of hypoventilation. About 90% of patients with OHS have concomitant OSA, defined as an apnea-hypopnea index (AHI) greater than 5 events per hour, and up to 70% with severe disease (AHI >30 events/h) [26–28].

UARS is a sleep-related breathing disorder, described by Guilleminault et al., in 1993, to identify patients who present increased respiratory effort and limited airflow during sleep, associated with increased upper airway resistance [29]. These patients usually complain of daytime sleepiness, fatigue, snoring, and difficulty staying asleep. Cognitive problems, headaches, anxiety, and irritability are also frequent. Physical examination revealed nasal obstruction, increased soft tissue, and craniofacial abnormalities associated with decreased upper airspace. The progression from UARS to OSA is debatable and there is no follow-up data to demonstrate the change in this condition. UARS in patients often go unrecognized and untreated. These patients arrive at the sleep clinic complaining of daytime sleepiness or fatigue and with a polysomnography examination that does not demonstrate the presence of OSA. The abnormalities frequently observed at polysomnography examination consist of periods of increased respiratory effort, disturbed sleep, the presence of respiratory events related to arousal (without oxygen desaturation), and flattening in the respiratory curve, which indicates limited airflow [30].

In general, sleep-related respiratory disorders can arise in NREM and REM sleep. However, in practice, we observe that many individuals present a worsening of respiratory events in REM sleep (due to muscle atony), maintaining more uniform breathing throughout the other sleep phases [31–33].

1.4 Further Reading

For an overview of sleep characteristics see Rowley (2012) [34]. Respiratory control and loop gain can be revised at Deacon-Diaz and Malhotra (2018) [13].

References

1. Huang W, Ramsey KM, Marcheva B, Bass J. Circadian rhythms, sleep, and metabolism. J Clin Invest. 2011;121(6):2133–41. https://doi.org/10.1172/JCI46043.
2. Zee PC, Turek FW. Sleep and health: everywhere and in both directions. Arch Intern Med. 2006;166(16):1686–8. https://doi.org/10.1001/archinte.166.16.1686.
3. Lee Y, Field JM, Sehgal A. Circadian rhythms, disease and chronotherapy. J Biol Rhythm. 2021;36(6):503–31. https://doi.org/10.1177/07487304211044301.
4. Meir Kryger TR, William C. Dement. Principles and practice of sleep medicine. 6th ed. Amsterdam: Elsevier; 2017.
5. Buchanan GF. Timing, sleep, and respiration in health and disease. Prog Mol Biol Transl Sci. 2013;119:191–219. https://doi.org/10.1016/B978-0-12-396971-2.00008-7.
6. Carley DW, Farabi SS. Physiology of sleep. Diabetes Spectr. 2016;29(1):5–9. https://doi.org/10.2337/diaspect.29.1.5.
7. Kryger M, Avidan A, Berry R. Atlas clínico de medicina do sono. 2nd ed. Amsterdam: Elsevier; 2015.
8. Bryant PA, Trinder J, Curtis N. Sick and tired: does sleep have a vital role in the immune system? Nat Rev Immunol. 2004;4(6):457–67. https://doi.org/10.1038/nri1369.
9. West JB. Respiratory physiology: the essentials. 9th ed. Philadelphia, PA: Lippincott Williams Wilkins/Wolters Kluwer Business; 2012.
10. Webster LR, Karan S. The physiology and maintenance of respiration: a narrative review. Pain Ther. 2020;9(2):467–86. https://doi.org/10.1007/s40122-020-00203-2.
11. Carroll JL, Agarwal A. Development of ventilatory control in infants. Paediatr Respir Rev. 2010;11(4):199–207. https://doi.org/10.1016/j.prrv.2010.06.002.
12. Berger KI, Ayappa I, Sorkin IB, Norman RG, Rapoport DM, Goldring RM. CO(2) homeostasis during periodic breathing in obstructive sleep apnea. J Appl Physiol. 1985;88(1):257–64. https://doi.org/10.1152/jappl.2000.88.1.257.
13. Deacon-Diaz N, Malhotra A. Inherent vs. induced loop gain abnormalities in obstructive sleep apnea. Front Neurol. 2018;9:896. https://doi.org/10.3389/fneur.2018.00896.
14. White DP. Pathogenesis of obstructive and central sleep apnea. Am J Respir Crit Care Med. 2005;172(11):1363–70. https://doi.org/10.1164/rccm.200412-1631SO.
15. Terziyski K, Draganova A. Central sleep apnea with Cheyne-stokes breathing in heart failure—from research to clinical practice and beyond. Adv Exp Med Biol. 2018;1067:327–51. https://doi.org/10.1007/5584_2018_146.
16. Hernandez AB, Patil SP. Pathophysiology of central sleep apneas. Sleep Breath. 2016;20(2):467–82. https://doi.org/10.1007/s11325-015-1290-z.
17. Nerbass FB, Piccin VS, Peruchi BB, Mortari DM, Ykeda DS, Mesquita FOS. Atuação da Fisioterapia no tratamento dos distúrbios respiratórios do sono. ASSOBRAFIR Ciência. 2015;6:23.
18. Sateia MJ. International classification of sleep disorders-third edition: highlights and modifications. Chest. 2014;146(5):1387–94. https://doi.org/10.1378/chest.14-0970.
19. Foldvary-Schaefer NR, Waters TE. Sleep-disordered breathing. Continuum (Minneap Minn). 2017;23(4):1093–116. https://doi.org/10.1212/01.CON.0000522245.13784.f6.

20. Berry RBBR, Gamaldo CE, Harding SM, Marcus CL, Vaughn BV, Tangredi MM, for the American Academy of Sleep Medicine. The AASM manual for the scoring of sleep and associated events: rules, terminology and technical specifications. Darien, IL: https://www.aasmnet.org; 2012.
21. Wellman A, White DP. Central sleep apnea and periodic breathing. In: Kryger M, Roth T, Dement W, editors. Principles and practice of sleep medicine. 5th ed. Amsterdam: Elsevier; 2010.
22. Berger M, Solelhac G, Horvath C, Heinzer R, Brill AK. Treatment-emergent central sleep apnea associated with non-positive airway pressure therapies in obstructive sleep apnea patients: a systematic review. Sleep Med Rev. 2021;58:101513. https://doi.org/10.1016/j.smrv.2021.101513.
23. Liu D, Armitstead J, Benjafield A, Shao S, Malhotra A, Cistulli PA, et al. Trajectories of emergent central sleep apnea during CPAP therapy. Chest. 2017;152(4):751–60. https://doi.org/10.1016/j.chest.2017.06.010.
24. Zeineddine S, Badr MS. Treatment-emergent central apnea. Chest. 2021;159:2449. https://doi.org/10.1016/j.chest.2021.01.036.
25. Zhang J, Wang L, Guo HJ, Wang Y, Cao J, Chen BY. Treatment-emergent central sleep apnea: a unique sleep-disordered breathing. Chin Med J. 2020;133(22):2721–30. https://doi.org/10.1097/CM9.0000000000001125.
26. Balachandran JS, Masa JF, Mokhlesi B. Obesity hypoventilation syndrome epidemiology and diagnosis. Sleep Med Clin. 2014;9(3):341–7. https://doi.org/10.1016/j.jsmc.2014.05.007.
27. Piper AJ. Nocturnal hypoventilation—identifying & treating syndromes. Indian J Med Res. 2010;131:350–65.
28. Lajoie AC, Kaminska M. Use of positive airway pressure in the treatment of hypoventilation. Sleep Med Clin. 2022;17(4):577–86. https://doi.org/10.1016/j.jsmc.2022.07.004.
29. Guilleminault C, Stoohs R, Clerk A, Cetel M, Maistros P. A cause of excessive daytime sleepiness. The upper airway resistance syndrome. Chest. 1993;104(3):781–7. https://doi.org/10.1378/chest.104.3.781.
30. Arnold WC, Guilleminault C. Upper airway resistance syndrome 2018: non-hypoxic sleep-disordered breathing. Expert Rev Respir Med. 2019;13(4):317–26. https://doi.org/10.1080/17476348.2019.1575731.
31. Alzoubaidi M, Mokhlesi B. Obstructive sleep apnea during rapid eye movement sleep: clinical relevance and therapeutic implications. Curr Opin Pulm Med. 2016;22(6):545–54. https://doi.org/10.1097/MCP.0000000000000319.
32. Kushida CA, Chediak A, Berry RB, Brown LK, Gozal D, Iber C, et al. Clinical guidelines for the manual titration of positive airway pressure in patients with obstructive sleep apnea. J Clin Sleep Med. 2008;4(2):157–71.
33. Peever J, Fuller PM. The biology of REM sleep. Curr Biol. 2017;27(22):R1237–R48. https://doi.org/10.1016/j.cub.2017.10.026.
34. Rowley JA, Badr MS. Normal Sleep. In: Badr MS, editor. Essentials of sleep medicine: an approach for clinical pulmonology. Totowa, NJ: Humana Press; 2012. p. 1–15.

Chapter 2
Positive Airway Pressure Treatment and Monitoring

2.1 Positive Airway Pressure Treatment

Obstructive sleep apnea (OSA) is defined as a condition in which repeated episodes of partial or complete airway obstruction occur during sleep. The body's response to blocked breath leads to brain arousal, sympathetic activation, and desaturation of oxygen in the blood. Repeated episodes of upper airway obstruction during sleep can cause sleep fragmentation and non-restorative sleep. Those who have OSA may complain of tiredness, excessive daytime sleepiness, insomnia, or morning headaches, but many are asymptomatic [1].

The main metric for diagnosing OSA is the apnea–hypopnea index (AHI) that reflects the average number of significant breathing disturbances per hour of sleep and is measured during some form of polysomnography (sleep study) [1]. Standard clinical practice to diagnose OSA requires a single overnight in-laboratory or in-home polysomnography or polygraphy study in which an AHI between 5 and 15 is classified as mild, 15–30 moderate, and more than 30 events/h as severe OSA [2]. The overall prevalence of any severity of OSA ranged from 9% to 38% in the general adult population (13–33% in men and 6–19% in women) and can be much higher in the elderly groups [1].

Until the early 1980s, the best-known treatment for obstructive sleep apnea syndrome with relevant symptoms (such as cardiac arrhythmia, pulmonary and systemic hypertension, morning headaches, polycythemia, etc.) was the tracheotomy procedure (which was maintained open only during sleep) [3]. It was in 1981 that Sullivan and collaborators published the first study showing the reversal of obstructive sleep apnea by using a positive pressure device applied through a nasal mask, during sleep [3]. The method, considered very simple at that time, proved to be remarkably effective, and since then positive pressure airway pressure (PAP) is the choice treatment for most sleep-related breathing disorders [4]. PAP may include continuous positive airway pressure (CPAP), bilevel PAP, auto-titrating PAP (APAP), and assisted servo-ventilation (ASV) (Table 2.1) [4].

V. S. Piccin, *Monitoring Positive Pressure Therapy in Sleep-Related Breathing Disorders*, https://doi.org/10.1007/978-3-031-50292-7_2

Table 2.1 Modes of positive airway pressure (PAP) [4]

Abbreviation	Mode	Mechanism of Action
CPAP	Constant positive airway pressure	Set pressure
Bilevel PAP	Bilevel positive airway pressure	Independently set inspiratory and expiratory pressures
APAP	Automatic positive airway pressure	Set range of pressures: Machine adjusts based on patient's breathing
ASV	Assisted servo-ventilation	Machine adjusts pressure based on minute ventilation: Rarely used for obstructive sleep apnea

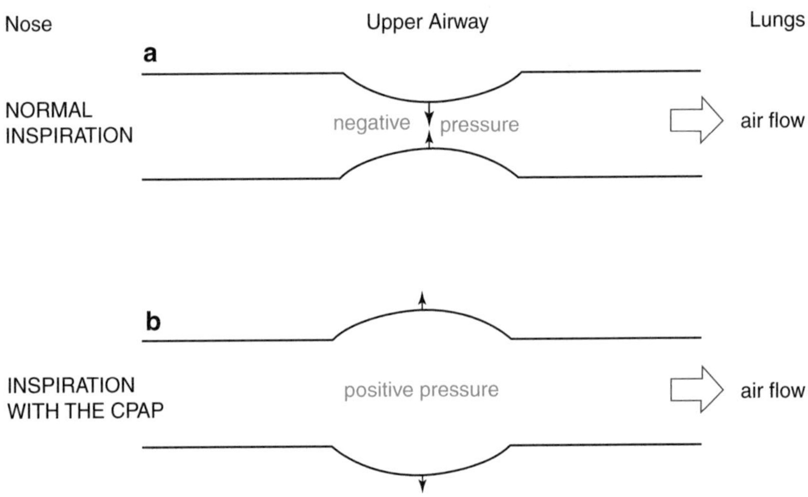

Fig. 2.1 Upper airway (UA) diagram showing the pneumatic support provided by CPAP. In normal inspiration (**a**), the pressure of the airflow is lower than the pressure on the tissues around the UA structure. Due to several factors (obesity, aging, etc.), UA can be less sustainable and collapse during sleep because of this differential pressure. The positive pressure generated by the CPAP (**b**) inside the UA acts as a pneumatic splint to support the upper airways during respiration, preventing its collapse. (Figure source: own work)

Presently, for OSA patients the most common treatment is the use of continuous positive airway pressure (CPAP), specially indicated for moderate and severe sleep apnea [5, 6]. CPAP has become the gold standard mainly due to its proven ability to improve ventilatory function [7], reduce symptoms such as excessive daytime sleepiness, and improve patients' quality of life [6].

CPAP therapy primarily works by providing a pneumatic splint to the muscular structure of the upper airway (UA), maintaining UA patency and preventing it from collapsing during the night (Fig. 2.1) [8]. Positive pressure is transmitted to the patient via nasal, oronasal, or facial (full face) interfaces throughout the breathing cycle (Fig. 2.2) [9].

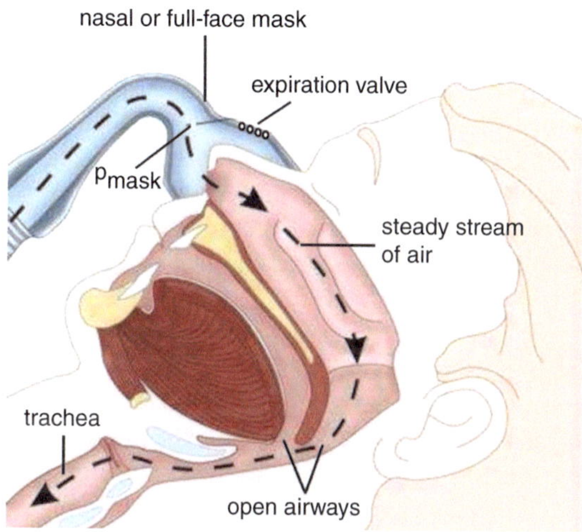

Fig. 2.2 Functionality of the CPAP therapy. The patient is connected to a CPAP device (through the mask) that generates a positive pressure to splint the upper respiratory tracts. (Source: Scheel et al. (2018), with permission [9])

However, patients suffering from obstructive apnea are not the only ones to benefit from CPAP. Also, for patients with predominant or partial manifestation of central sleep apnea (CSA) during the night, associated with multiple etiologies, the initial treatment of choice, according to the recommendations of the American Academy of Sleep Medicine, is the CPAP [10].

In fact, most CSA etiologies respond favorably to CPAP, particularly CSA associated with OSA, although the largest body of evidence supporting CPAP use in the CSA has been from studies in CHF patients. Specifically, a group of researchers from the University of Toronto (Ontario, Canada) demonstrated that congestive heart failure (CHF) patients show improvement in morbidity and mortality when using CPAP with fixed pressure and residual apnea–hypopnea index below 15 events per each hour of sleep (CANPAP study) [11].

Patients with idiopathic CSA have also shown improved treatment with CPAP, even in the absence of concurrent OSA. This effect is particularly pronounced in supine-dependent CSA, to avoid ventilatory overshoot caused by a primary restrictive respiratory event, and as consequence leading to the occurrence of central apnea [10].

In addition to CPAP, the bilevel pressure machine has also been shown to be effective in treating sleep-disordered breathing [5, 12]. The bilevel positive pressure device maintains two pressure levels during respiratory cycle: the IPAP (inspiratory airway pressure or inspiratory pressure) and the EPAP (expiratory airway pressure or expiratory pressure) that are configured independently. The differential between these two pressure levels, also called ventilatory delta or support pressure, already gave the bilevel device important applications in the health area, mainly for those patients in need of ventilatory support. In the sleep-disordered breathing field, bilevel can be indicated in cases of obesity hypoventilation syndrome plus OSA, congenital alveolar hypoventilation syndrome, patients with pulmonary ventilatory disorders associated with OSA, and for those OSA patients who have not adhered to CPAP or for cases in which the indicated CPAP pressure is too high [5, 8, 12].

CPAP and bilevel pressure therapy can be offered in two modalities, fixed pressure or variable pressure, commonly called automatic CPAP (APAP) and automatic bilevel, respectively [8]. The automatic devices have sensors that detect a reduction in the respiratory flow curve, changing the pressure level to maintain the permeability of the UA [13]. During sleep, there is a gradual decrease in muscle activity and a consequent increase in intraluminal negative pressure, which favors instability and UA collapse. Conversely, the genioglossus muscle has mechanoreceptors that respond to negative pressure in the pharynx, when there is an obstructive respiratory event, leading to a reflex action of this dilating muscle and stabilizing the airway. The algorithm of the automatic devices considers this variation in muscle tone during sleep, increasing or decreasing the pressure to reach the lowest and most effective treatment pressure, generating greater comfort for the patient during the sleep. In the specific case of automatic bilevel machines, the automatic EPAP adjustment occurs to prevent apneas, and the automatic IPAP adjustment acts to prevent the occurrence of hypopneas. Automatic bilevel devices can act in two ways: with fixed EPAP and self-adjusting IPAP, or with both, self-adjusting EPAP and IPAP according to each manufacturer's algorithm.

2.2 Positive Airway Pressure Adherence

Adherence to PAP devices is one of the determining factors for treatment success of sleep-disordered breathing [14]. Many factors influence this process, such as marital status, age, chosen interface, anatomy of the upper airway, race, and socioeconomic factors [15–17].

Studies show that the results of the first week of PAP use are determinants of long-term success [18]. Factors such as high AHI, higher oxygen desaturation, higher daytime sleepiness, lower number of adverse effects, family support, and educational interventions proved to be predictors of good adherence [18, 19].

The main beneficial intervention in the PAP adherence process is patient follow-up. We highlight the regular visits with a qualified professional, the education of the patient and companion regarding OSA, and the ease of professional–patient contact at the beginning of the adaptation process, for quick interventions if necessary [20].

Aiming to improve comfort and adherence to PAP, manufacturers have been developing new comfort technologies such as expiratory pressure relief, pressure ramp with automatic adjustment, humidification system, among others [8]. About expiratory relief, the objective is to minimize airflow resistance during expiration, and this function can be graduated according to patient comfort. Regarding the automatic ramp, the software detects a decrease in airflow at the beginning of CPAP use and immediately increases the ramp pressure until UA stabilizes. But there is no evidence in the literature that the use of comfort functions improves adherence to PAP [8, 21]. Also, it is important to point out that some patients report improvement

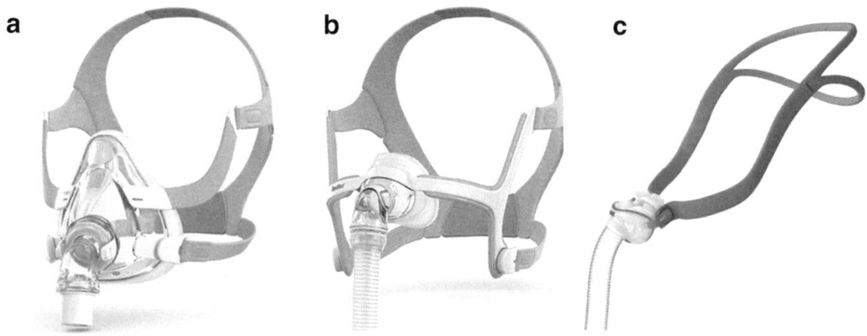

Fig. 2.3 (**a**) AirFit F20 oronasal mask from ResMed; (**b**) AirFit N20 nasal mask from ResMed; (**c**) AirFit P10 pillow mask from ResMed. (Image courtesy of Dr. Vivien Schmeling Piccin)

after adjusting comfort functions, but others may be less able to tolerate it (such as pressure variations in the exhalation relief function or pressure changes at superficial phase of sleep in the automatic ramp) and have worse sleep quality.

Conversely, for the PAP adherence process to be successful, the proper interface choice is fundamental [8, 22]. There are several models and types of interfaces available on the market, including nasal and oronasal masks and intranasal pillows (Fig. 2.3). Nasal masks should be the first choice in the fitting process [17]. Nasal mask requires less pressure to open the airway when compared to oronasal masks, improves sleep quality, and is related to greater adherence to positive pressure treatment. Moreover, the nasal mask (including pillow interfaces) is also better tolerated by patients [22, 23].

2.3 Patient Monitoring

One of the major challenges for the effectiveness of the treatment of sleep-related breathing disorders is the low adherence to PAP. About 29–83% of patients use PAP less than 4 hours per night. Nowadays we know that using positive pressure equipment for a short period of time is better than not using the device, and the longer the equipment is used at night, the more health and quality of life are benefiting. We call these time-dependent benefits. In general, the first week predicts long-term use and symptomatic patients are the most predisposed to adhere. Educational interventions, follow-up, intensive support, and quickly resolving problems related to the use of PAP can help to improve adherence [8].

We must be careful when starting the process of PAP adherence, because depending on previous experience and prejudice, PAP acceptance may not be so positive. We must explain to the patient what the disease is about, what were the clinical implications of sleep respiratory disturbances and emphasize the treatment benefit on health and quality of life.

During PAP therapy follow-up, we must periodically reassess the patient, considering the data obtained from the device and the patient's own reports about improvement in their symptoms or any difficulties observed. Difficulties wearing the PAP mask, dry mouth/throat, difficulty to exhale, claustrophobia, facial pain due to mask pressure, noise, irritation/skin injury, air leaks, headaches, dry eyes, aerophagia, etc. are difficulties usually reported by patients who start pressure therapy. But even before waiting for the patient's report, countless data can be obtained by remote monitoring systems. This gives the health professional the possibility of a quick intervention to encourage the patient's adherence to the treatment.

Several systems for monitoring the use of positive pressure therapy are available on the market. By means of an internal sensor in the PAP device, these systems can demonstrate the residual AHI (apnea–hypopnea index), the effective time of PAP use, mask leaks, types of respiratory events, signs of respiratory flow and PAP pressure, triggering of the equipment when in automatic mode, among others (Table 2.2) [24].

The data found in the segment reports must be carefully assessed. A high rate of residual apnea–hypopnea may mean that the pressure level of the equipment is inadequate to eliminate respiratory events. Conversely, it can also indicate the presence of respiratory events of central origin (which may be resolved over time or require the recommendation of another type of equipment to resolve it—such as, for example, a bilevel device).

Table 2.2 Examples of positive pressure therapy data, obtained by the device's monitoring system

Manufacturer	Data
All	Patient and device characterization Report period Therapeutic mode (CPAP or bilevel, fixed, or automatic pressure) Pressure relief Ramp time (automatic or fixed, time in minutes) Device pressure Intentional/unintentional leak Residual AHI Time (average and median) of PAP use per night Number of nights that the PAP was (and was not) in use Percentage of nights the PAP was used ≥4 hrs/night
Intentional/unintentional leak according to some manufacturers	
Philips Respironics	It allows the description of two types of leaks on the report: Total (intentional + unintentional) or unintentional. For all PAP devices, leak values below 60 L/min is accepted Above 60 L/min of leaks, the algorithm does not recognize the patient's respiratory flow. If the automatic switch-off function is active, in the event of a high leak, the therapeutic pressure starts to decrease and after 3 min the device switches off automatically. Without the automatic shutdown function active, excessive leaks will appear in the bar graph in black
ResMed	Displays unintentional leak values. In general, leak values below 24 L/min are accepted on CPAP devices when using a mask with an exclusively nasal route and 36 L/min with an oronasal route. ResMed system's equipment used in the sleep field can maintain therapeutic pressure to a significantly higher leak (approximately 60 L/min) at the expense of the device's engine effort

Table 2.2 (continued)

Manufacturer	Data
Fisher & Paykel	Sum of intentional and unintentional leaks. In general, the CPAP works well at leak values below 60 L/min (for nasal masks, and 80 L/min for oronasal masks). In F&P reports, it is important to correct excessive leaks for a period greater than 30% of CPAP use

Important tips

Intentional leak means the expected leak that occurs at the mask exhalation port. Unintentional leak means the unexpected leak that occurs generally by improper adjustment of the mask on the patient's face, or leakage through the mouth

PAP: Positive pressure in the upper airway; CPAP: Continuous positive pressure on the upper airway; bilevel: Bilevel positive airway pressure (bilevel) machines have two different pressures: a higher pressure when breathing in (IPAP) and a lower pressure when breathing out (EPAP).

Some important clarifications about data that are presented in the reports:

- Maximum value: Represents the highest value achieved during treatment
- Median: Represents the intermediate number of a classified list of numbers. Half the numbers in the list are lower and half the numbers are greater (e.g., 3, 3, 4, 5, 5, 5, 6, 9, 12, 23, 48: Median = 5). The median reduces the impact of extreme values to a minimum and better represents the group of values. The average hours of use (therapy) are calculated in relation to the PAP days of use
- Percentile: Represents that, in a certain percentage of the time (90% or 95%, according to the manufacturer), the variable (e.g., pressure) is in that value or below it. Similarly, in a certain percentage of the remaining time (10% or 5%, according to the manufacturer), the variable is above that value

2.4 Telemonitoring

The health system is currently facing new challenges (such as world population growth, increased longevity, chronic diseases, etc.). Today, we face a crisis in the healthcare system to meet the needs of patients and control excessive medical expenses. In this context, telemedicine promotes remote medical care through technology, streamlines the delivery of medical care, increases patient access to health care, and saves time and costs.

Patients with sleep-related respiratory disorders often require prompt interventions to improve PAP adherence. However, these interventions can generate high costs for the health system, such as expenses related to health specialist outpatient services and patient displacement. In this regard, advances in telemedicine have shown potential solutions for patient follow-up and care, effectively improving adherence at a lower cost.

New positive pressure equipment for treating sleep-related breathing disorders allows therapeutic data to be verified remotely, using the Internet, by sending data via a cell phone module, Bluetooth, or downloading an SD card to the user's computer. CPAP tracking systems are built with connectivity to allow remote access, providing information about daily use, pattern of use, respiratory events (residual AHI), type of residual events (central, obstructive), mask leaks, and CPAP pressure. Data is transferred every day and is available via a central secured data center (cloud) for healthcare providers/professionals or, for some devices, via an application, accessed directly by the patient, to stimulate self-management. This data allows the health professional to readjust parameters, suggest solutions, refer them to other specialists for combination therapies, and even change therapeutic strategies (Fig. 2.4) [25, 26].

Although studies indicate improved adherence to PAP therapy with the use of a telemonitoring system, there is still no concise literature data on this subject, neither for adults nor children [27]. What exists is a consensus among sleep professionals that these systems are effective in monitoring patients who have already incorporated the use of positive pressure equipment in their routine. Perhaps the greatest difficulty regarding the use of these monitoring instruments is the lack of standardization of the information generated by the different manufacturers, which impairs interpretation of the data obtained. One example is the information about an air leak through the interface which, for certain manufacturers, is presented by the sum of the intentional and unintentional leaks and in others just the value of unintentional leaks is presented. Another example is that every CPAP device manufacturer uses a proprietary algorithm to detect, classify, and aggregate events throughout the night to finally compute for physicians a brand specific residual AHI. The types of residual events included in the summary of nightly events vary between CPAP manufacturers essentially by including or not central hypopneas and respiratory effort-related arousals (RERAs) [28]. Not knowing these differences (and many more) leads to misinterpretation of usage data and can negatively influence the strategies adopted for patient treatment.

Conversely, the lack of in-depth research on the effectiveness of monitoring systems for monitoring positive pressure therapy makes the use of the information

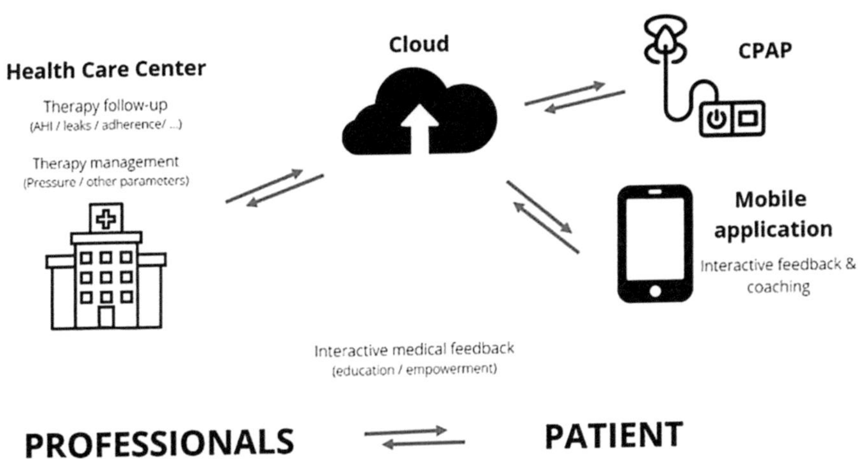

Fig. 2.4 Interactions between patients and healthcare professionals in telemonitored CPAP-treated OSA patients. *CPAP* continuous positive airway pressure, *OSA* obstructive sleep apnea. (Source: Dusart, C et al. (2022), under the terms and conditions of the Attribution 4.0 International (CC BY 4.0) [29])

generated empirical, in addition to being extremely dependent on the experience of the professional in the field.

2.5 Ethical Concerns

Integrating technology and medicine, such as electronic medical records and telemonitoring, has the potential to enhance healthcare quality. However, it also raises questions about patient privacy. To address privacy concerns, it is important to ensure transparency regarding patient adherence to any digital system and data-sharing policies. One way to improve patients' awareness of the data obtained through positive pressure equipment is to inform them adequately about sharing pressure therapy use data with members of the multidisciplinary sleep team or using it for academic or research purposes. When requesting consent for data extraction, healthcare professionals must ensure that patients receive adequate informed consent about what aspects of their information are being used. Maintaining transparency between patients, providers, and healthcare institutions is crucial. This can be achieved through dynamic consent solutions or informed consent approaches that facilitate seamless and streamlined engagement and communication between individuals and those who use their data. Furthermore, healthcare professionals must comply with legal and ethical regulations when storing and sharing patient data across different jurisdictions [30, 31].

2.6 Further Reading

PAP technologies are treated in depth in the book: Advances in the Diagnosis and Treatment of Sleep Apnea (series title: Advances in Experimental Medicine and Biology—doi.org/10.1007/978-3-031-06413-5). This is an ideal book for health professionals who are interested in learning about the latest technologies in treating and diagnosing sleep apnea.

References

1. Senaratna CV, Perret JL, Lodge CJ, Lowe AJ, Campbell BE, Matheson MC, et al. Prevalence of obstructive sleep apnea in the general population: a systematic review. Sleep Med Rev. 2017;34:70–81. https://doi.org/10.1016/j.smrv.2016.07.002.
2. Lechat B, Naik G, Reynolds A, Aishah A, Scott H, Loffler KA, et al. Multinight prevalence, variability, and diagnostic misclassification of obstructive sleep apnea. Am J Respir Crit Care Med. 2022;205(5):563–9. https://doi.org/10.1164/rccm.202107-1761OC.
3. Sullivan CE, Issa FG, Berthon-Jones M, Eves L. Reversal of obstructive sleep apnoea by continuous positive airway pressure applied through the nares. Lancet. 1981;1(8225):862–5.

4. Feinsilver SH. Obstructive sleep apnea: treatment with positive airway pressure. Clin Geriatr Med. 2021;37(3):417–27. https://doi.org/10.1016/j.cger.2021.04.004.
5. Kushida CA, Littner MR, Hirshkowitz M, Morgenthaler TI, Alessi CA, Bailey D, et al. Practice parameters for the use of continuous and bilevel positive airway pressure devices to treat adult patients with sleep-related breathing disorders. Sleep. 2006;29(3):375–80.
6. Kakkar RK, Berry RB. Positive airway pressure treatment for obstructive sleep apnea. Chest. 2007;132(3):1057–72. https://doi.org/10.1378/chest.06-2432.
7. Berthon-Jones M, Sullivan CE. Time course of change in ventilatory response to CO2 with long-term CPAP therapy for obstructive sleep apnea. Am Rev Respir Dis. 1987;135(1):144–7. https://doi.org/10.1164/arrd.1987.135.1.144.
8. Piccin VS, de Pressão A, Positiva A. Cuidados e Segmento. In: Sono. vol Série atualização e reciclagem em pneumologia—SPPT. São Paulo: Editora Atheneu; 2017.
9. Scheel M, Berndt A, Simanski O. Application of Kalman filter for breathing effort reconstruction for OSAS patients in breathing therapy. Automatisierungstechnik. 2018;66(12):1064–71. https://doi.org/10.1515/auto-2018-0067.
10. Ginter G, Badr MS. Central sleep apnea. Handb Clin Neurol. 2022;189:93–103. https://doi.org/10.1016/B978-0-323-91532-8.00011-2.
11. Arzt M, Floras JS, Logan AG, Kimoff RJ, Series F, Morrison D, et al. Suppression of central sleep apnea by continuous positive airway pressure and transplant-free survival in heart failure: a post hoc analysis of the Canadian continuous positive airway pressure for patients with central sleep apnea and heart failure trial (CANPAP). Circulation. 2007;115(25):3173–80. https://doi.org/10.1161/circulationaha.106.683482.
12. Schäfer H, Ewig S, Hasper E, Lüderitz B. Failure of CPAP therapy in obstructive sleep apnoea syndrome: predictive factors and treatment with bilevel-positive airway pressure. Respir Med. 1998;92(2):208–15.
13. Morgenthaler TI, Aurora RN, Brown T, Zak R, Alessi C, Boehlecke B, et al. Practice parameters for the use of autotitrating continuous positive airway pressure devices for titrating pressures and treating adult patients with obstructive sleep apnea syndrome: an update for 2007. An American Academy of sleep medicine report. Sleep. 2008;31(1):141–7.
14. Weaver TE. Adherence to positive airway pressure therapy. Curr Opin Pulm Med. 2006;12(6):409–13. https://doi.org/10.1097/01.mcp.0000245715.97256.32.
15. Jacobsen AR, Eriksen F, Hansen RW, Erlandsen M, Thorup L, Damgård MB, et al. Determinants for adherence to continuous positive airway pressure therapy in obstructive sleep apnea. PLoS One. 2017;12(12):e0189614. https://doi.org/10.1371/journal.pone.0189614.
16. Billings ME, Auckley D, Benca R, Foldvary-Schaefer N, Iber C, Redline S, et al. Race and residential socioeconomics as predictors of CPAP adherence. Sleep. 2011;34(12):1653–8. https://doi.org/10.5665/sleep.1428.
17. Andrade RG, Piccin VS, Nascimento JA, Viana FM, Genta PR, Lorenzi-Filho G. Impact of the type of mask on the effectiveness of and adherence to continuous positive airway pressure treatment for obstructive sleep apnea. J Bras Pneumol. 2014;40(6):658–68. https://doi.org/10.1590/S1806-37132014000600010.
18. Weaver TE, Grunstein RR. Adherence to continuous positive airway pressure therapy: the challenge to effective treatment. Proc Am Thorac Soc. 2008;5(2):173–8. https://doi.org/10.1513/pats.200708-119MG.
19. Sawyer AM, Gooneratne NS, Marcus CL, Ofer D, Richards KC, Weaver TE. A systematic review of CPAP adherence across age groups: clinical and empiric insights for developing CPAP adherence interventions. Sleep Med Rev. 2011;15(6):343–56. https://doi.org/10.1016/j.smrv.2011.01.003.
20. Holmdahl C, Schöllin IL, Alton M, Nilsson K. CPAP treatment in obstructive sleep apnoea: a randomised, controlled trial of follow-up with a focus on patient satisfaction. Sleep Med. 2009;10(8):869–74. https://doi.org/10.1016/j.sleep.2008.08.008.

21. Kushida CA, Berry RB, Blau A, Crabtree T, Fietze I, Kryger MH, et al. Positive airway pressure initiation: a randomized controlled trial to assess the impact of therapy mode and titration process on efficacy, adherence, and outcomes. Sleep. 2011;34(8):1083–92. https://doi.org/10.5665/SLEEP.1166.
22. Dibra MN, Berry RB, Wagner MH. Treatment of obstructive sleep apnea: choosing the best Interface. Sleep Med Clin. 2017;12(4):543–9. https://doi.org/10.1016/j.jsmc.2017.07.004.
23. BaHammam AS, Singh T, George S, Acosta KL, Barataman K, Gacuan DE. Choosing the right interface for positive airway pressure therapy in patients with obstructive sleep apnea. Sleep Breath. 2017;21(3):569–75. https://doi.org/10.1007/s11325-017-1490-9.
24. LILD M-F, Piccin VS. Dispositivos de Terapia com Pressão Positiva (PAP) e Interpretação de Relatórios. In: Manual de Métodos Diagnósticos em Medicina do Sono. Rio De Janeiro: Editora Atheneu. Série SONO; 2018.
25. Hwang D, Chang JW, Benjafield AV, Crocker ME, Kelly C, Becker KA, et al. Effect of telemedicine education and telemonitoring on CPAP adherence: the tele-OSA randomized trial. Am J Respir Crit Care Med. 2017;97(1):117–26. https://doi.org/10.1164/rccm.201703-0582OC.
26. Hwang D. Monitoring progress and adherence with positive airway pressure therapy for obstructive sleep apnea: the roles of telemedicine and mobile health applications. Sleep Med Clin. 2016;11(2):161–71. https://doi.org/10.1016/j.jsmc.2016.01.008.
27. Contal O, Poncin W, Vaudan S, De Lys A, Takahashi H, Bochet S, et al. One-year adherence to continuous positive airway pressure with telemonitoring in sleep apnea hypopnea syndrome: a randomized controlled trial. Front Med (Lausanne). 2021;8:626361. https://doi.org/10.3389/fmed.2021.626361.
28. Midelet A, Borel JC, Tamisier R, Le Hy R, Schaeffer MC, Daabek N, et al. Apnea-hypopnea index supplied by CPAP devices: time for standardization? Sleep Med. 2021;81:120–2. https://doi.org/10.1016/j.sleep.2021.02.019.
29. Dusart C, Andre S, Mettay T, Bruyneel M. Telemonitoring for the follow-up of obstructive sleep apnea patients treated with CPAP: accuracy and impact on therapy. Sensors (Basel). 2022;22(7):2782. https://doi.org/10.3390/s22072782.
30. Chiruvella V, Guddati AK. Ethical issues in patient data ownership. Interact J Med Res. 2021;10(2):e22269. https://doi.org/10.2196/22269.
31. Fields BG. Regulatory, legal, and ethical considerations of telemedicine. Sleep Med Clin. 2020;15(3):409–16. https://doi.org/10.1016/j.jsmc.2020.06.004.

Chapter 3
Respiratory Flow Curve

3.1 The Importance of Assessing Respiratory Flow Patterns During Sleep

While assessing compliance and treatment parameters through the respiratory flow curve on the device's statistical report, it is important to note that certain criteria were arbitrarily defined. These criteria include a residual Apnea-Hypopnea Index (AHI) of less than 5 events per hour of sleep, a mean daily usage of the positive airway pressure (PAP) therapy device equal to or greater than 4 hours per night, and the use of PAP therapy for 4 hours/night at least 70% of the evaluated period [1]. Despite the arbitrary nature of these criteria, they serve as the standard measures guiding our perception of therapeutic success when monitoring a patient using positive pressure therapy to treat sleep-related breathing disorders (SRBD). It is worth noting that even though we are aware of the time-dependent benefits of PAP therapy [2], these defined parameters remain a key instrument in assessing therapeutic outcomes.

In most cases, data from statistical reports will be sufficient to ensure proper patient follow-up. However, in certain patients, we will find that additional information will be extremely relevant for adequate and effective positive pressure treatment.

Who are those patients? They are those patients who are OSA diagnosed but started to present central sleep apnea at PAP therapy; or patients with respiratory central events where the events distribution in the course of the night can guide treatment options, among many other situations in which we will need additional information during the PAP use for adequately guide SRBD treatment [3].

For these challenging patients, the respiratory flow curve signal will provide lots of information on the breathing pattern during sleep and will even provide us with precious clues for therapeutic conduct. For example, previous studies have shown that visual airflow waveform morphology is a helpful parameter for identifying wakefulness at sleep (Fig. 3.1) and this is a helpful information to investigate those

V. S. Piccin, *Monitoring Positive Pressure Therapy in Sleep-Related Breathing Disorders*, https://doi.org/10.1007/978-3-031-50292-7_3

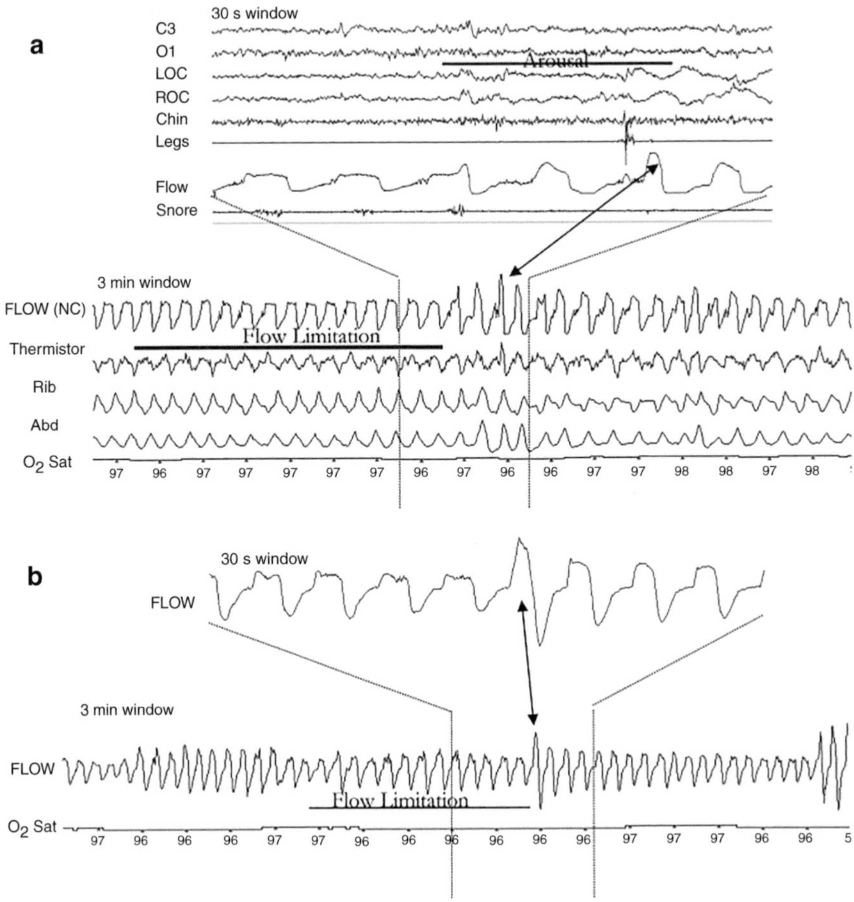

Figure 3.1 (**a**) The nasal flow signal, especially the large inspiratory amplitude after signs of flow restriction, can be a very useful tool to identify awakenings (i.e., it is a signal that could replace the electroencephalographic signal to identify awakenings during sleep). Sample signal display used for scoring of full nocturnal polysomnography with all signals visible. (**b**) Sample view of screen used to score respiratory events using the flow signal and oximetry alone. *LOC* refers to left outer canthus; *ROC* right outer canthus, *NC* nasal cannula, *Abd* abdomen. (Source: Modified after Ayappa et al., 2004 (with permission))

individuals who present residual drowsiness, despite presenting adequate data of PAP usage in the device statistical report [4, 5]. Also studies have also shown that a sequence of breaths with flattened inspiratory flow/time contour (suggesting events of flow limitation) usually terminate in arousal and have autonomic consequences like apneas [6].

Moreover, respiratory flow curve structure can not only indicate the occurrence of arousals, but also regular breathing pattern, periods of limited respiratory flow, snoring, and even some oral expiration events (Fig. 3.2) [3, 4].

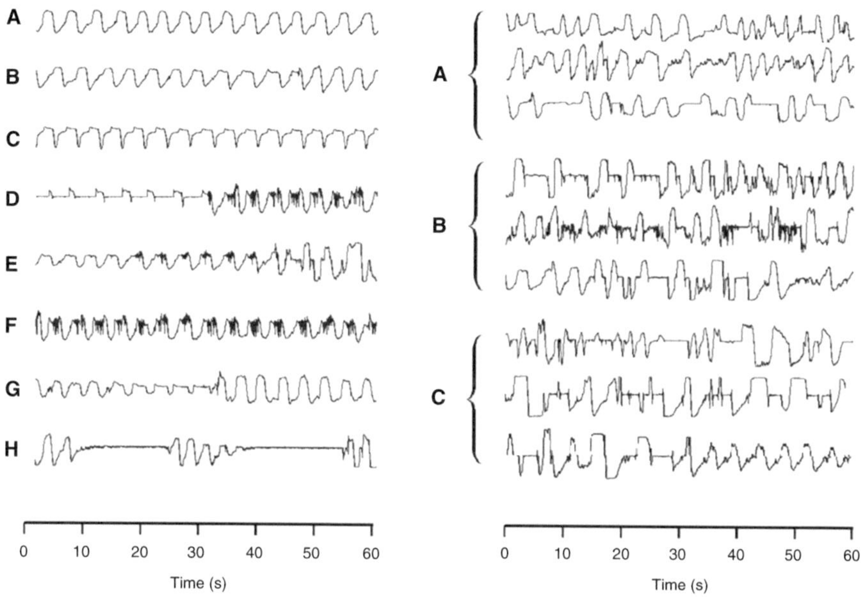

Fig. 3.2 Sleep and wakefulness respiratory flow characteristics (sleep and wakefulness morphology criteria). The flow signal was assessed in arbitrary units on nasal prongs. (Source: Modified after Guerrero et al., 2010 (with permission))

3.2 How Flow Curves Are Generated

Breath detection is essential in sleep and respiratory physiology research and in several clinical settings. Despite its significance, detecting respiration is technically difficult. Physiological events such as sighs, swallows, transient reductions and pauses (hypopneas and apneas) in breathing during sleep recordings, as well as measurement artifacts including signal drift, EKG artifact, electrical noise on the airflow signal, and mask leaks, each present unique challenges when attempting to quantify breath timing accurately [7].

In the field of sleep, to quantify key respiratory variables such as maximum inspiratory flow, flow disturbance, or flow limitation, precise identification of inspiration and exhalation is required. Manual detection and calculation of respiratory parameters takes time and is potentially subject to human error and not practical for large data sets. Therefore, several algorithms have been developed for automatic respiratory detection. Most use an airflow signal, a volume signal, or both, and apply different threshold criteria to identify breaths [7].

Modern CPAP devices are sensitive to variations in pressure due to inspiratory and expiratory movements during respiration (Fig. 3.3). These fluctuations are captured by a flow sensor located inside the PAP device. By means of an analysis of the pressure sensor, the resultant electrical signal derives the airflow signal. After a drift correction, carried out by the device software (using algorithms specific to each manufacturer), we can visualize a graphical reproduction of the respiratory flow curve.

The quality of the represented respiratory flow curve will depend on the quality of the equipment that is producing it, mainly its capacity for amplification and linearization of the acquired signals, and its sampling rate. In general, amplification systems inserted in devices that provide the respiratory flow curve (such as polysomnography equipment, mechanical ventilation devices, among others) may use alternating current (AC) or direct current (DC) inputs, that will work differently with signals time constancy. Typically, PAP devices for sleep-related respiratory disorders use DC inputs. By using adequate filters signal interference is minimized (Fig. 3.4) [8].

The linearization of signals concerns the filters used (e.g., high- and low-frequency filters). The purpose of the filter is to suppress undesirable signals from the signal we are measuring. It is a conditioning method of the signals obtained [9]. For example, a signal that usually interferes with the airflow derivation signal is the heart rate pulse signal, which has a higher frequency than the respiration rate. The application of a low-pass filter reduces this interference and provides a better definition of the resulting signal [10]. However, it is important to note that accurate visualization of the flow contour by nasal cannula/pressure transducer can be compromised by over-filtering. Sampling rate (number of values per second

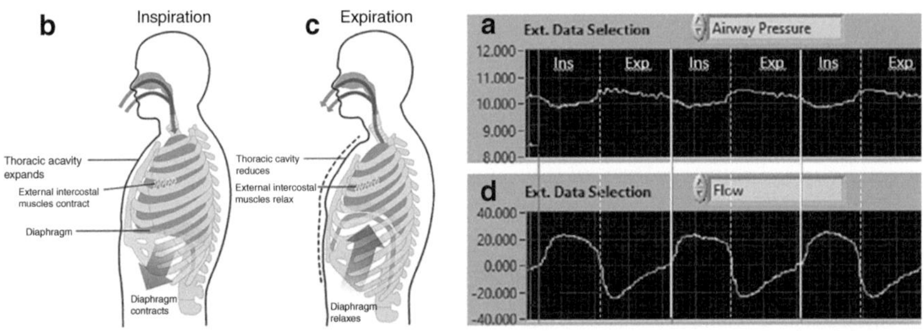

Fig. 3.3 The pressure curve (**a**) shows a small variation in inspiration (**b**) and expiration (**c**) due to the respiratory movement performed by the individual (action of the respiratory muscles). (**d**) Respiratory flow curve. (Source: Modified after ©2316 Inspiration and Expiration by https://openstax.org CC BY-SA 4.0)

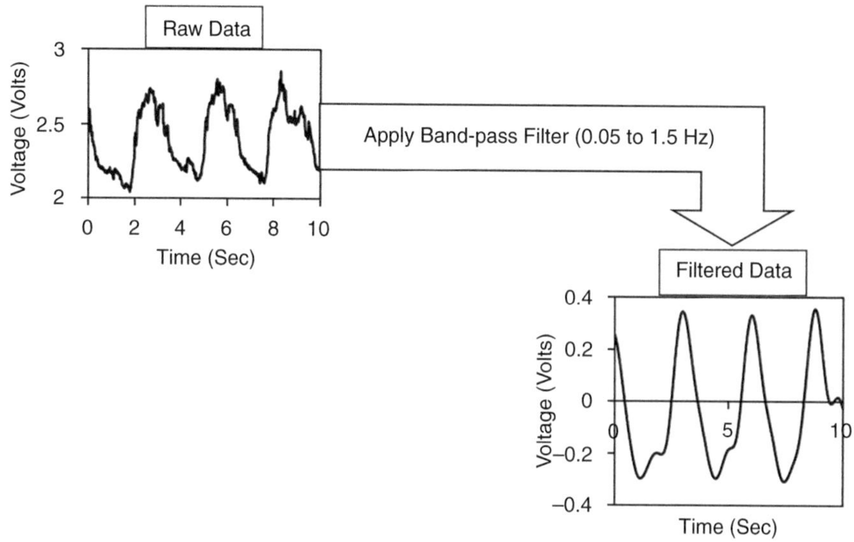

Fig. 3.4 Respiration frequency raw data at sampling frequency of 100 Hz (Raw Data) and the same respirations frequency after treatment with band-pass filter (Filtered Data). (Modified after Al-Halhouli et al., 2021 (with permission))

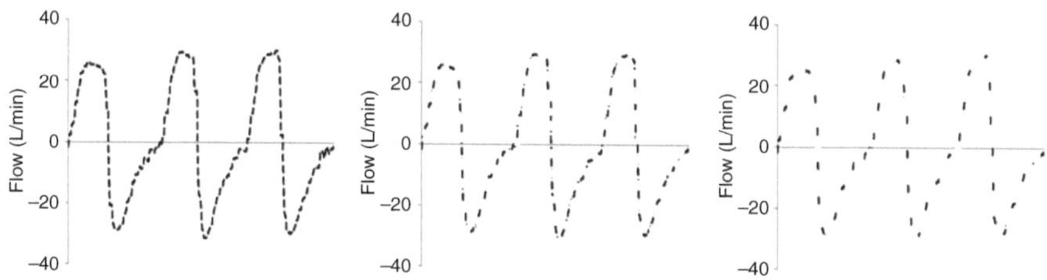

Fig. 3.5 Schematic example of different sampling rates (from left to right, starting with the highest and progressing to the lowest sampling rate), and how different sampling rates will represent the same respiratory flow curve by plotting data. (Figure source: own work)

(described in Hertz) that are stored to represent the signal) should be at least 100 hZ to obtain accurate flow contour as has been described in the AASM scoring manual [11].

Specifically in relation to the sampling rate of the respiratory signal, sophisticated sensors will provide a much more detailed airflow curve (much more "points" to represent the flow curve in a given period of time). More modest sensors will provide a simplified flow curve (fewer representative "points" to derivate the flow curve over a period of time), but it can still be representative for respiratory pattern analysis (Fig. 3.5). In general, the airway flow curve does not require a very high sampling rate. A sampling rate of approximately 10–50 Hz is sufficient to interpret the airflow signals.

3.3 Downloading Airflow Curves

Nowadays, many manufacturers allow healthcare providers to view detailed airflow data. The most popular are ResMed, Philips Respironics, and Fisher & Paykel Healthcare. Whereas Philips Respironics and Fischer & Paykel Healthcare already have detailed automatic download graphic data in the download factory settings, the ResMed equipment must be configured. This is due to the fact that the ResMed data contains more graphic data than other manufacturers. Thus, to preserve the memory of the professional's computer, this data will only be downloaded with some download configuration.

In this book, we focus on the high-resolution graphic data of ResMed PAP devices for sleep-related respiratory disorders. With an understanding of the detailed graphs presented by the ResMed PAP devices, the graphical interpretation of other manufacturers should not be difficult.

For advanced graphical assessment of ResMed positive pressure machines for sleep-related respiratory disorders, you will need the ResScan™ software.

ResScan™ is ResMed's PC-based clinical analysis and patient data management software that allows you to update device therapy parameters and download, analyze, and store treatment data. It takes a deeper look into patient therapy data using detailed graphs and reports, allowing you to review therapy breath-by-breath across a number of therapy metrics (including AHI, leak, and pressure information) in order to gain clinical insights to improve therapy, enhance efficacy, and support long-term compliance.

ResScan™ allows the tracking of long-term clinical and compliance trends using summary graphs and allows the review of device settings and key clinical indices via easy-to-read statistics. Compatible with most ResMed therapy devices, ResScan™ data can be collected via the data card or USB, according to the device. In addition, you can modify the therapy settings on all non-life assistance devices.

You can find information on how to install ResScan™ software in the clinical menu on ResMed's own website.

3.4 Important Tips for Managing Flow Curve Analysis Software

When opening the ResScan™ program on your computer, note that the ResScan™ 6.0 version or higher incorporated a security step in accessing patient data (Fig. 3.6). The login and password required are the same as those used for accessing Windows on your computer. If you have no Windows user access, you can create one by following the instructions at https://support.microsoft.com/pt-br/help/13951/windows-create-user-account. Use the same registered Windows and user password for the ResScan™ program. An alternative access option would be to right-click and access the ResScan™ program icon as an administrator (Fig. 3.7).

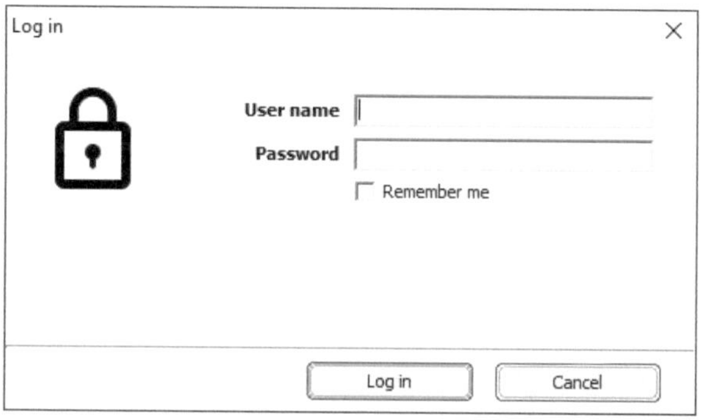

Fig. 3.6 When the ResScan™ program is installed on your computer, after opening the program this window immediately appears. Use the same login and password that you already use on your computer to access Windows. (Figure Copyright ResMed (with permission))

After accessing ResScan™ program, insert the PAP device SD card into the reader, and create a new patient or open an existing patient file where you want to transfer the data (Fig. 3.8) and click on "Download data" (Fig. 3.9). Then click "Select" on the data line (Fig. 3.10). This is where you will modify the options to upload data in high resolution. Without this option correctly configured, it is not possible to visualize the respiratory flow curve and other advanced charts. It is important to note that if you have previously downloaded patient data without these settings, you will not be able to view the high-resolution information prior to the appropriate download settings.

In the "Download Data" window, choose "All data in summary" to set the period of interest. The period of interest is the number of nights you want to download the high-resolution data (Fig. 3.11). Also check the box for "Include equivalent number of high frequency data sessions".

Remember that the more nights you select, the more space you will occupy in your computer's memory (five nights of evaluation are generally sufficient for a good understanding of the patient's breathing pattern during sleep). Based on the device model and software version, up to 30 most recent detailed data sessions can be available. If you want to adjust these download options for all patients, instead to have to configure the advanced data option every time you download the patient's data card, check the "Set these as my default options" box.

After these configuration settings, click on the "Ok" button and click on the "Start Download" option. Once the download has completed, click on the "Close" button. From then on you will be able to view the home screen of the patient's folder, with the left side panel showing the dates when the positive pressure equipment was used (and the availability of advanced data on specific dates) (Fig. 3.12).

Although the ResScan™ software presents several possibilities for managing high-resolution graphical data, we will focus on visualizing and analyzing respiratory flow curves in this book. The evaluation of the respiratory flow curve is our goal. As already mentioned, several other manufacturers also allow the visualization of this data, an important management tool for patients who use positive airway pressure devices for sleep-disordered breathing treatment.

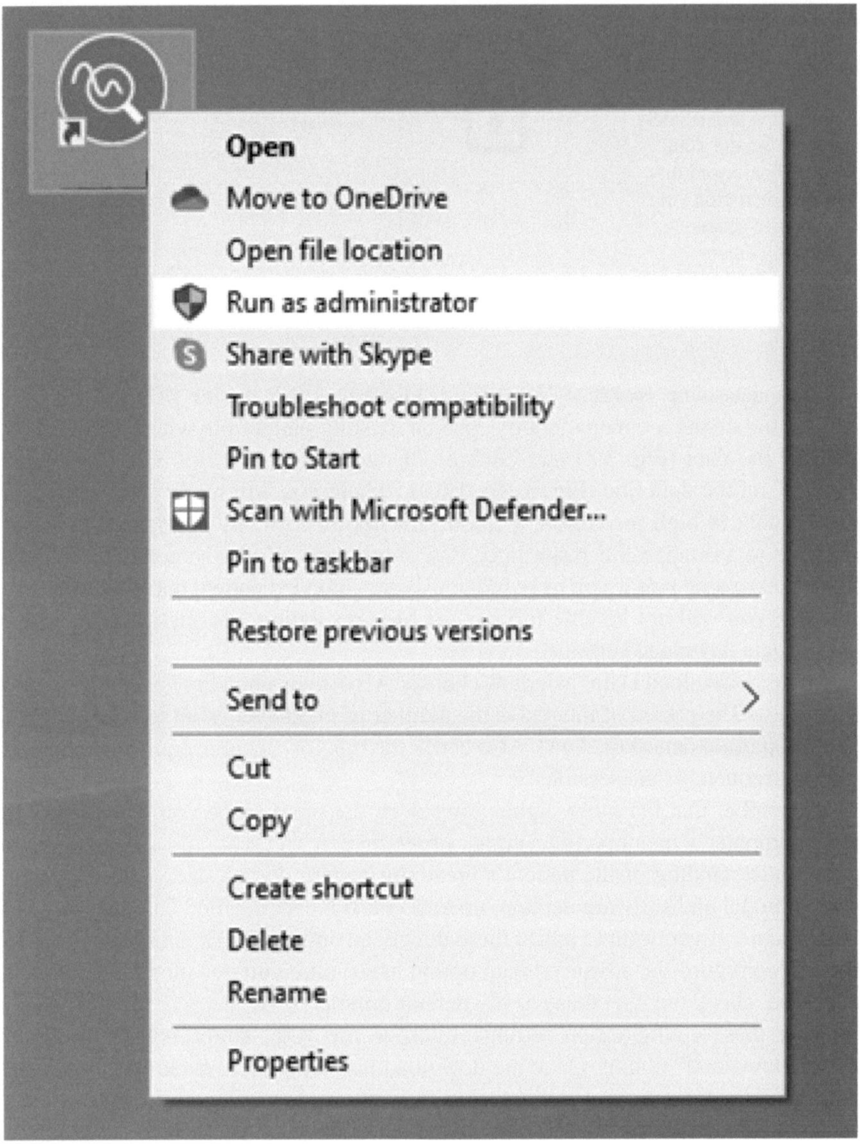

Fig. 3.7 This is an option to access the ResScan™ program if you do not have a password to access as a Windows user. Right click on the ResScan™ program icon and access it as an administrator. (Figure courtesy from Dr. Vivien Schmeling Piccin)

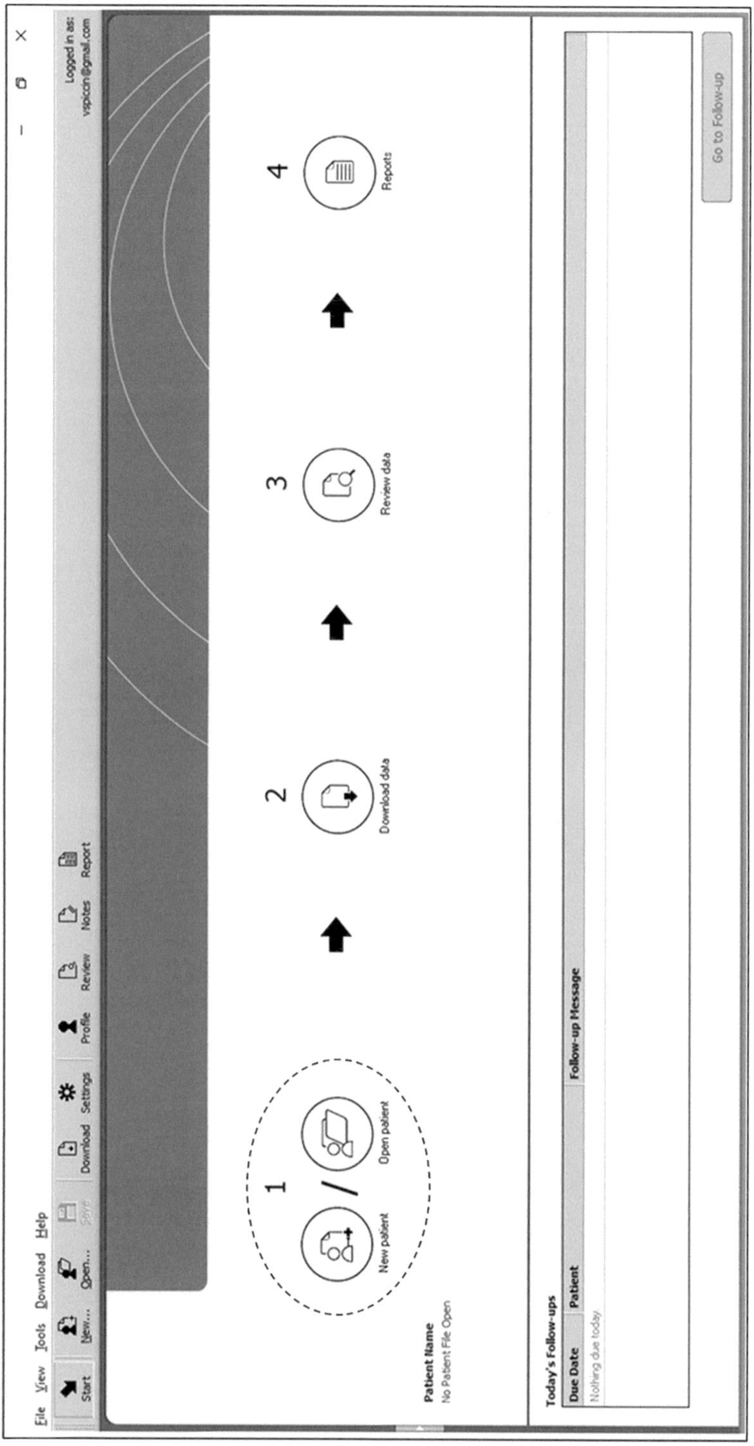

Fig. 3.8 ResMed's ResScan™ home screen. Open or create a new patient by clicking on the first icon "New patient/Open patient" (dotted circle). (Figure Copyright ResMed (with permission))

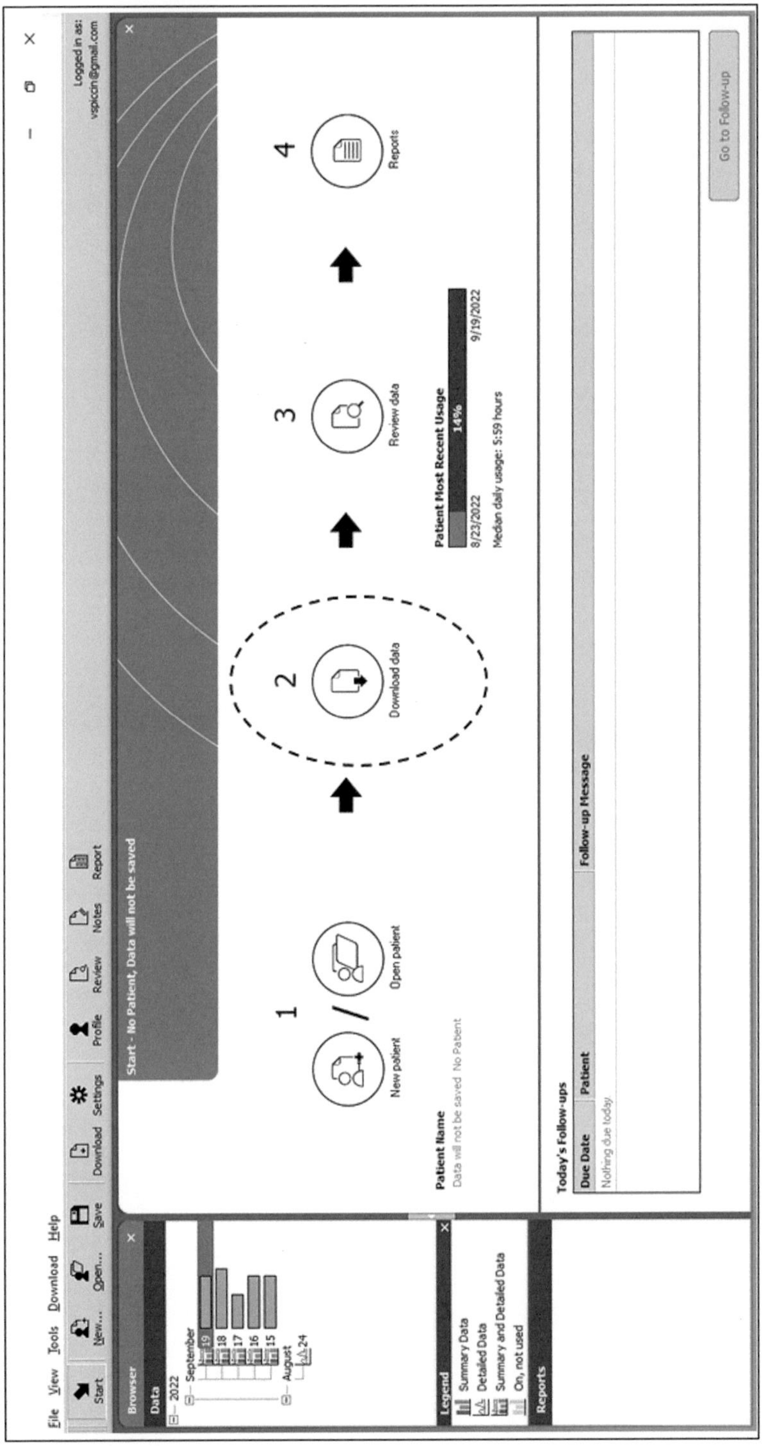

Fig. 3.9 ResMed's ResScan™ "Download data" screen. Download data by clicking on the second icon (dotted circle). (Figure Copyright ResMed (with permission))

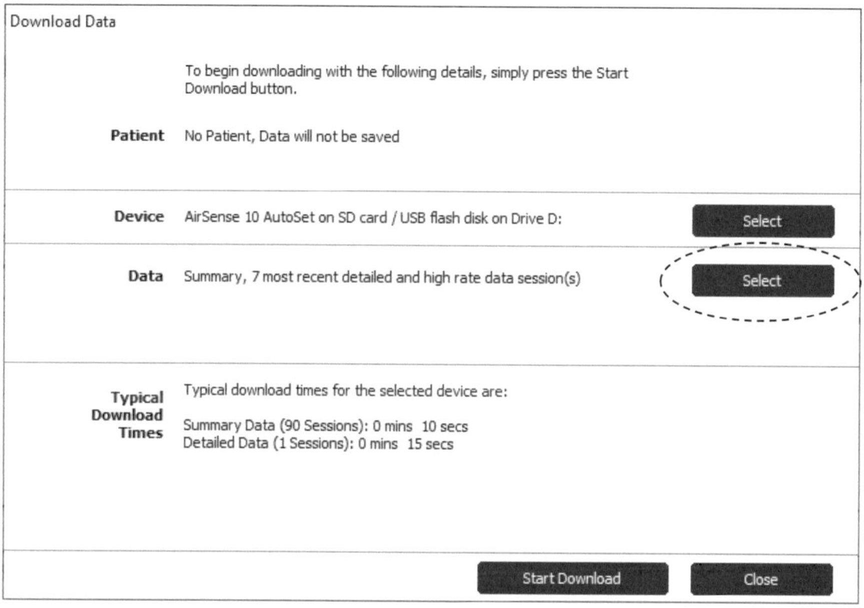

Fig. 3.10 Under "Data", click the "Select" option (dotted circle). This is where you will edit the options for downloading data in high resolution. Without this option properly configured, it is not possible to view the respiratory flow curve. (Figure Copyright ResMed (with permission))

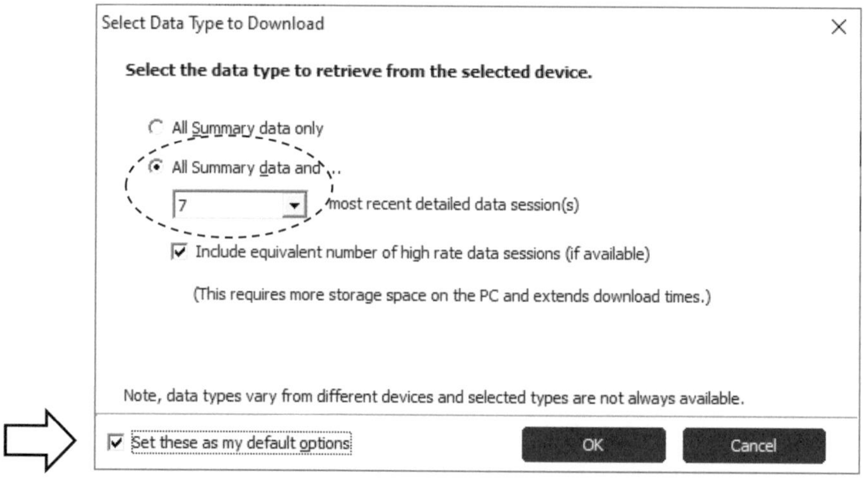

Fig. 3.11 Select here how many nights you want to view high-resolution data and check the box of an equivalent number of high-rate data sessions (dotted circle). If you want this download setting to be permanently on your computer, click on "Set these options as default option" (arrow). By clicking that option, it will not be necessary to configure the advanced data option every time you download the patient's data card. (Figure Copyright ResMed (with permission))

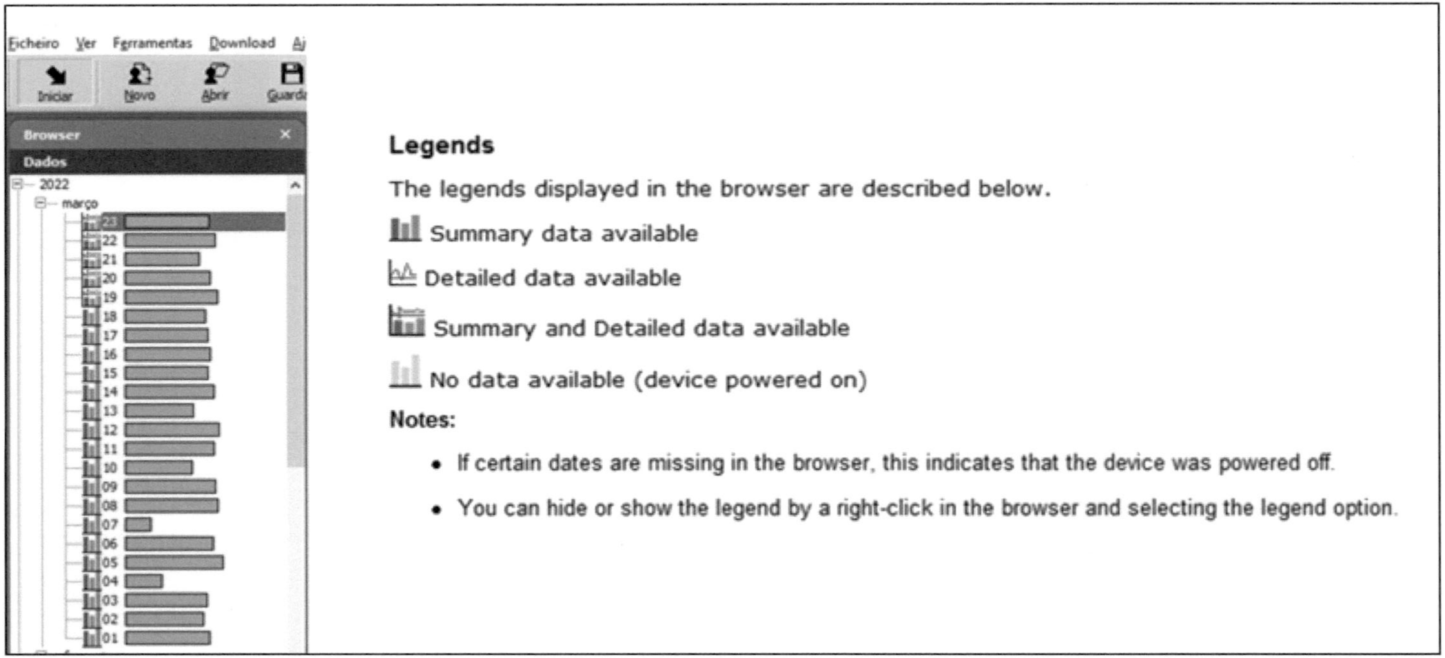

Fig. 3.12 Detail of the left side panel of the patient's folder, showing the dates when the positive pressure equipment was used and the availability of advanced data on specific dates. On the right side, we describe the legends of the figures displayed in the browser. (Figure Copyright ResMed (with permission))

3.5 Working with Detailed Graphs

In ResScan™ software, in the patient's folder (left window), click on the date you want to see the detailed respiratory airflow graph. Next, in the right pane, click "Detailed Graphs" and "Click to load detailed data" (Fig. 3.13). After that, click on the graph options icon (Fig. 3.14). In the graph options icon, you can select the information you want to view on the "Navigation" screen and on the "Detailed" screen.

In the graph options, you define the plots you want to display in the upper window ("Navigation") as well as in the lower window of the screen ("Detailed") (Fig. 3.15). Make sure the number of graphs that are visible at once is the same number of plots that you set previously.

After defining the information to be displayed in the "Navigation" and "Detail" windows, select the time interval on which you wish to center your evaluation (Fig. 3.16). Normally, in the Navigation window, we set the visualization of the data for the whole night (approximately 8 or 10 hours). In the Detailed window, visualization in the 5-minute interval allows a good graphical evaluation of the respiratory flow curve.

Graphic curves can be organized in multiple ways for better visualization (e.g., respiratory events under respiratory flow). To do this, use your mouse cursor on the right side of the graphic curve you want to change position; when a "little hand" icon appears, click, hold, and drag the graph curve up or down (Fig. 3.17).

You can also control the view scale, which is displayed on the left side of the plot window. To change the scales, use your mouse cursor on the left side (at the top of the graph scale), click, hold, and drag the graph scale up or down. In addition, arrows on the right side of the screen will pop up when you drag the cursor to that screen position. Use these arrows to help centralize the graphs in the window (Fig. 3.18).

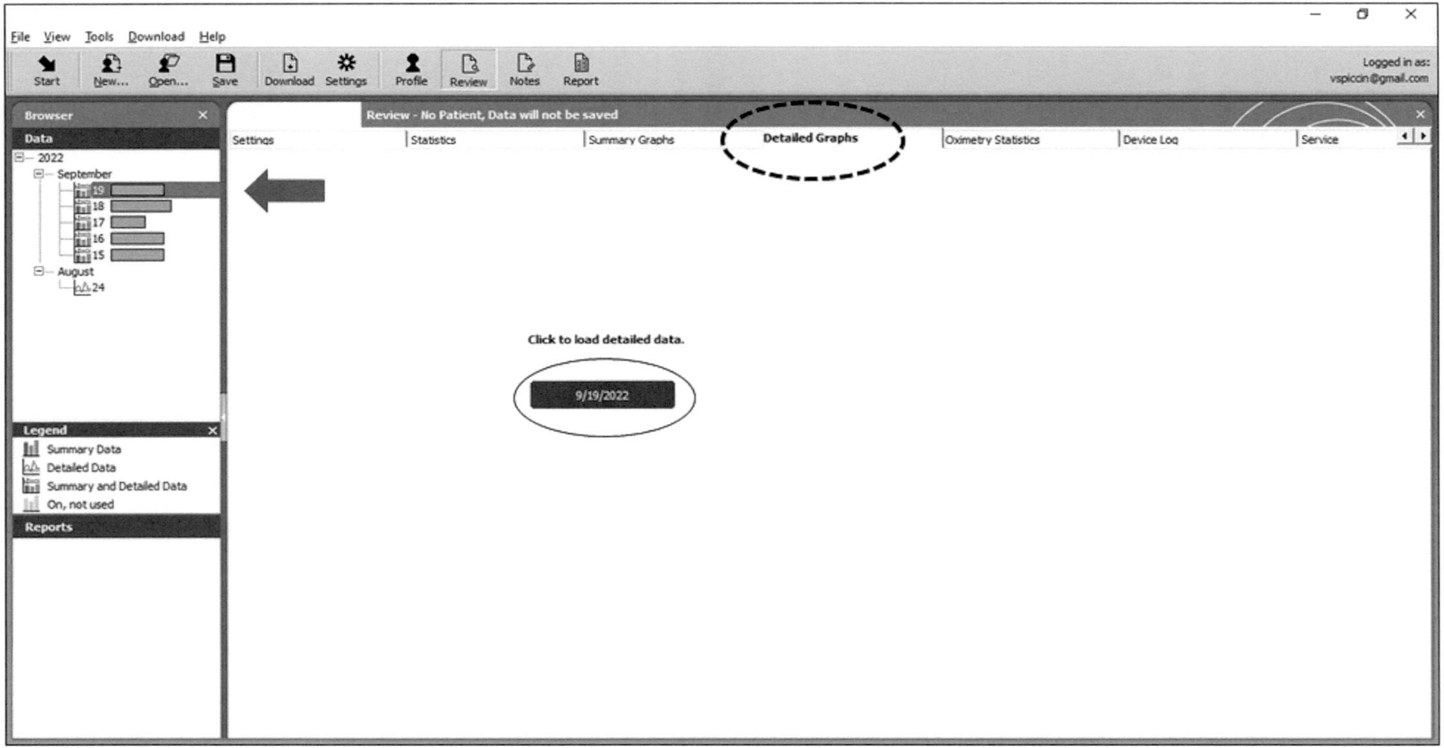

Fig. 3.13 Specifying an assessment date of detailed graph data on the ResScan™ screen. Select the date you would like to see the detailed respiratory airflow graph (arrow). Then, on the right window click on "Detailed Graphs" option (dotted circle) and "Click to load detailed data" (close circle). (Figure Copyright ResMed (with permission))

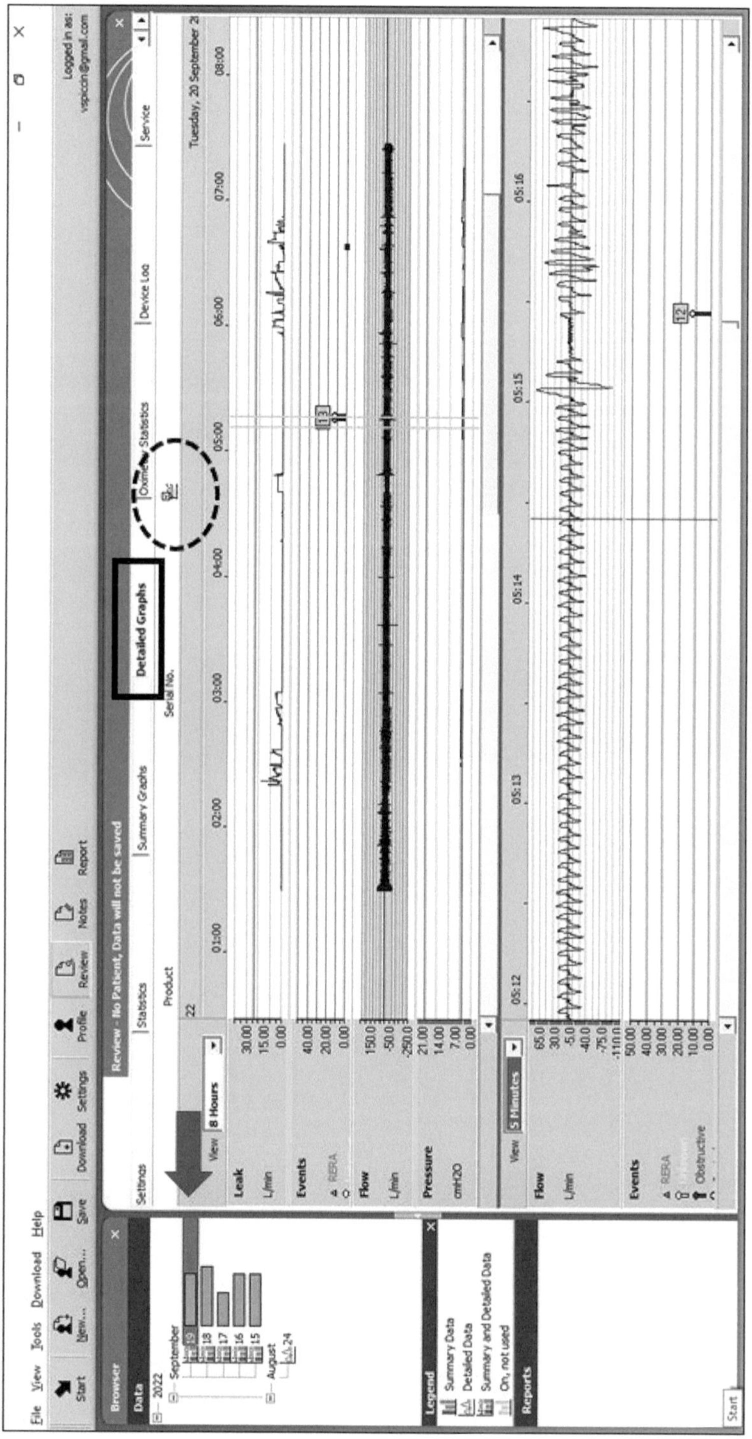

Fig. 3.14 In the graph options icon (dotted circle), you can select what information you want to see on the "Navigation" screen and on the "Detailed" screen. (Figure Copyright ResMed (with permission))

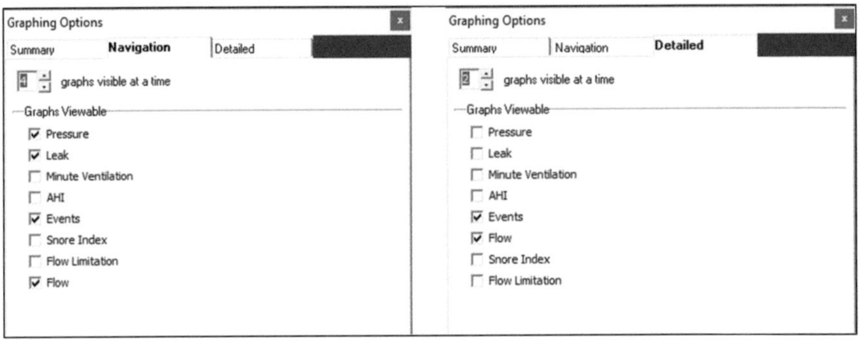

Fig. 3.15 In this figure, we can see the information options on the navigation screen as well on the detailed screen. These options vary based on the type of equipment. For bilevel equipment, there are more options (such as, e.g., inspiratory/expiratory time ratio, or even oxygen and pulse saturation data when oximeter is coupling at the positive airway pressure device). Make sure the number of "Graphs visible at a time" is the same number of plots as you previously have defined. (Figure Copyright ResMed (with permission))

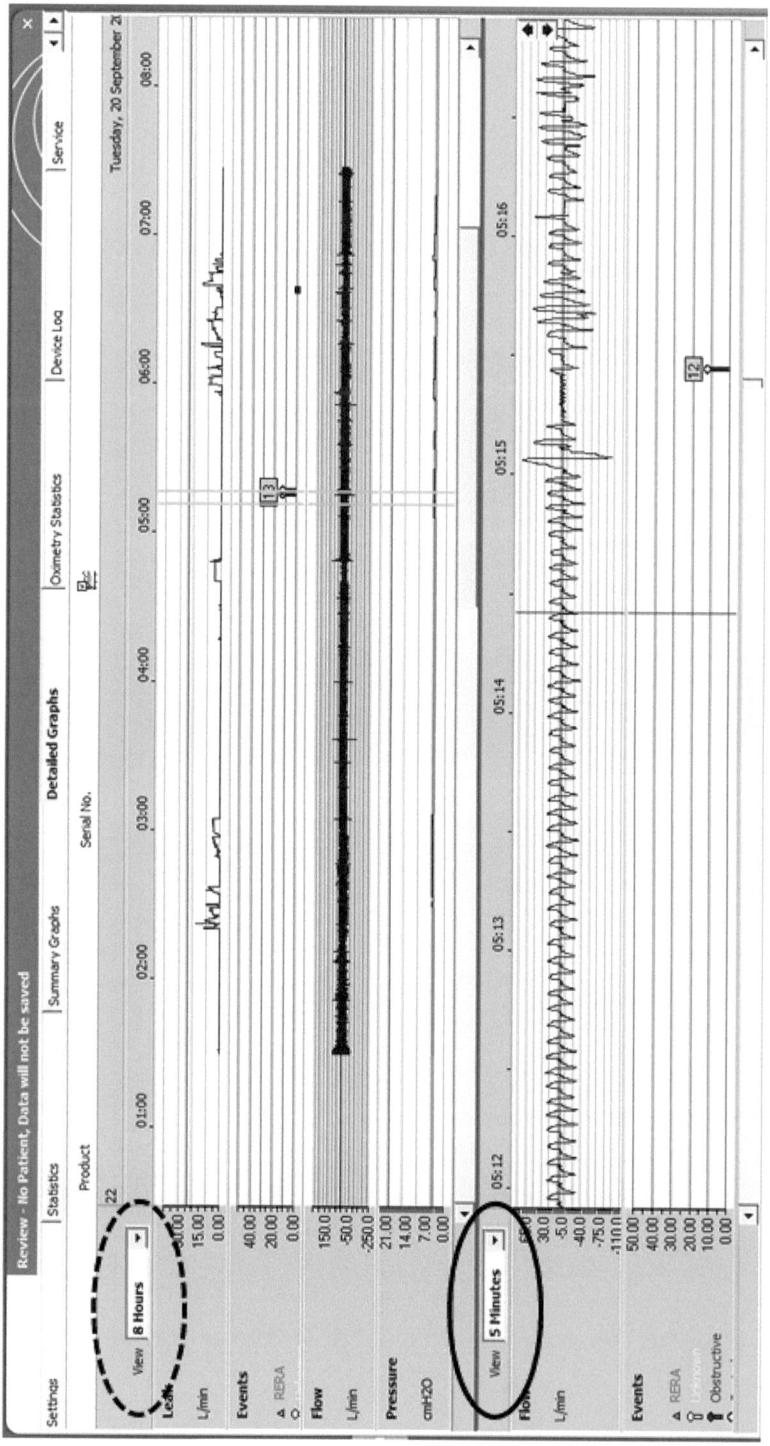

Fig. 3.16 Normally, in the Navigation window, we define the data visualization for the entire night (approximately 8- or 10-hour window). In the Detailed window, visualization in the 5-minute window time interval allows a good respiratory flow curve graphical assessment. (Figure source: own work)

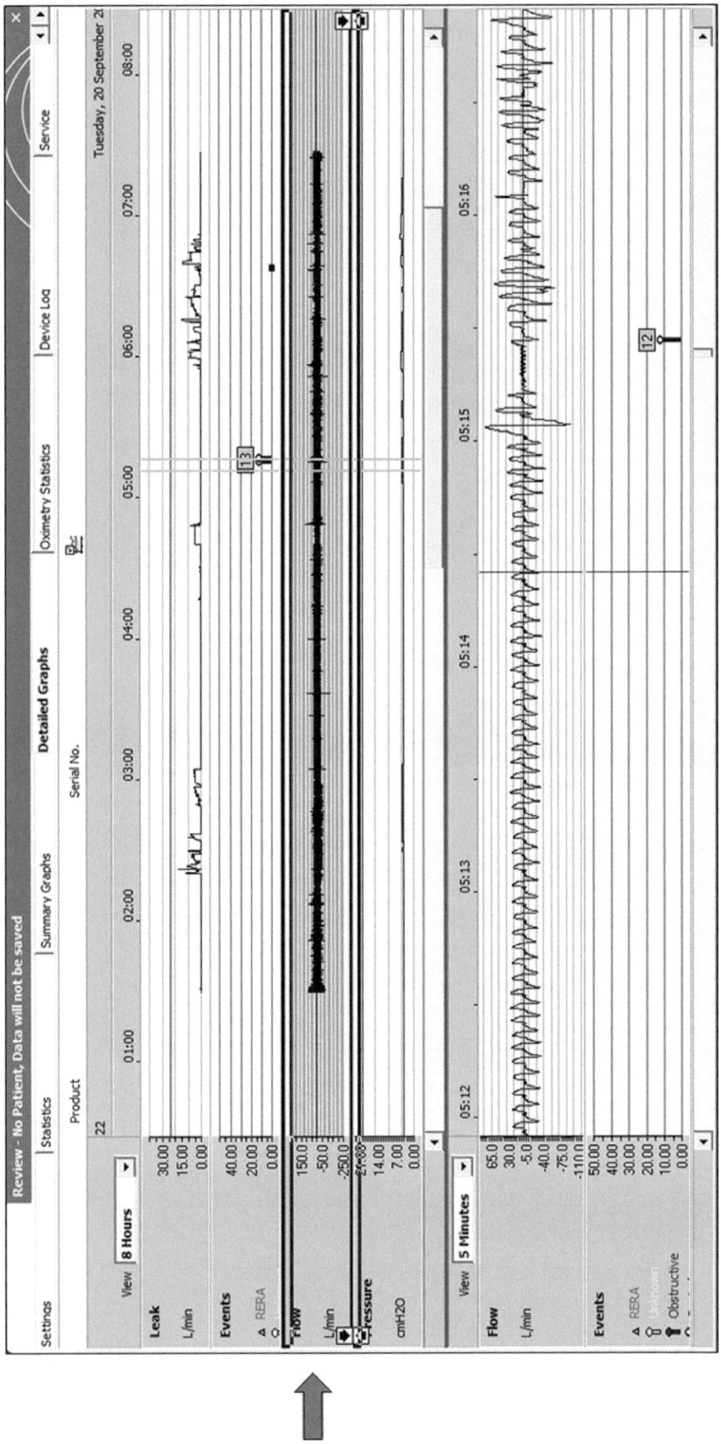

Fig. 3.17 Use your mouse cursor on the right side of the graphic curve you want to change position; when a "little hand" icon appears (not shown in this figure), click, hold, and drag the graph curve up or down. (Figure source: own work)

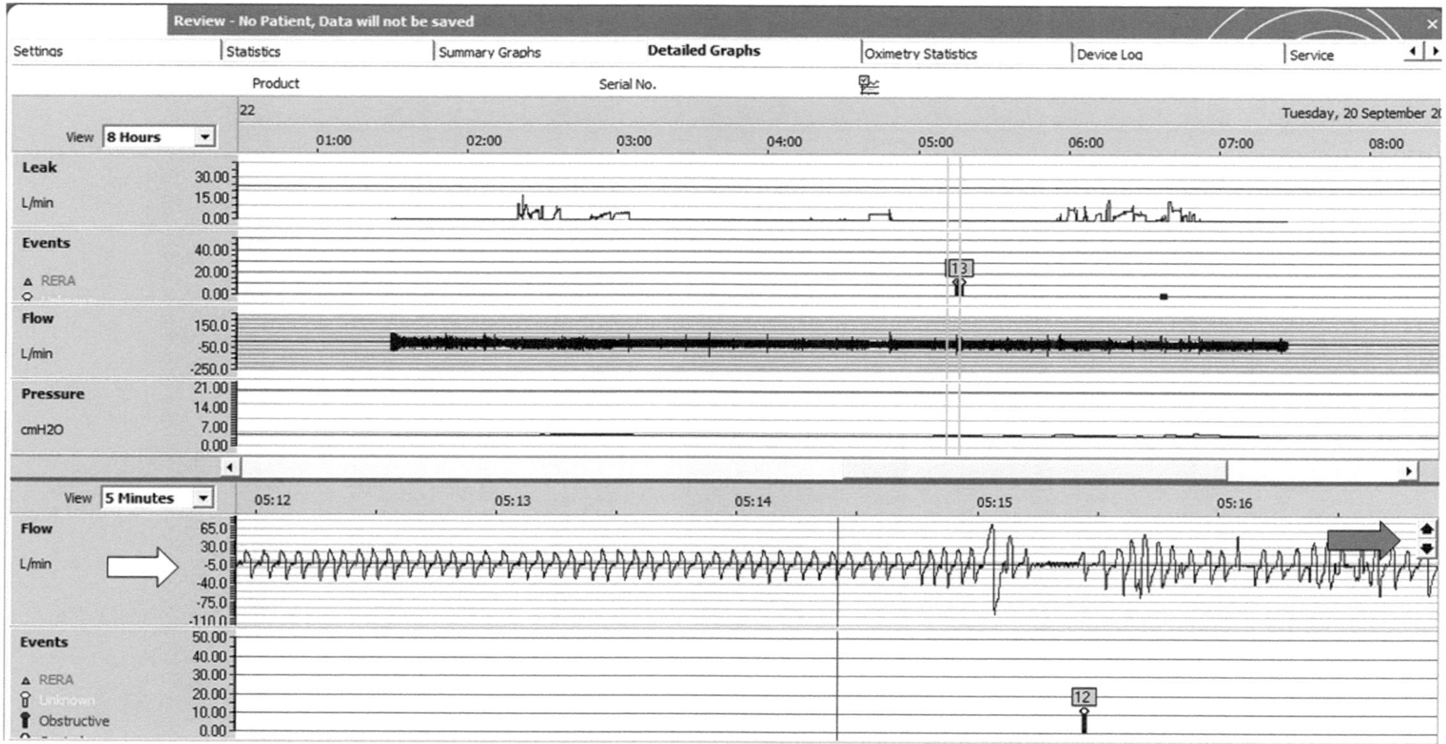

Fig. 3.18 To change scales, use your mouse cursor on the left side (on top of the graphic scale), click, hold, and drag the graph scale up or down (white arrow). Also, arrows on the right side of the screen will appear when you drag the cursor to this screen position. Use these arrows to better centralize the plots on the window (gray arrow). (Figure source: own work)

3.6 How to Share Detailed Graph Data

Often, evaluation of the patient's PAP therapy outcome must be discussed in a group of specialists, especially when we are dealing with more challenging patients. Not all team members work in the same physical space or even in the same town or country. In such cases, the high-definition graphic data can be shared. The professional with the original data can zip the file and send it to their colleagues. The one who receives the data will be able to visualize all the details by following the steps indicated here.

3.6.1 Sending Data to Healthcare Professionals

Firstly, locate the computer's root folder: OS (C:) (Fig. 3.19).

In the OS (C:) folder, locate the "Users" folder (Fig. 3.20). In the "Users" folder, locate the "Public" - "Public Documents" - "ResMed" - "ResScan" - "Patients" folder. In the "Patients" folder, locate the patient's folder.

Open the patient's folder, select everything that is on that folder, compress the file (using .zip or .rar), and send this compressed file by e-mail using a large data file upload tool (i.e., Dropbox, Google Drive, etc.) (Fig. 3.21). A tip that will make it easier for your colleague who will receive this file is to name the compressed file with the surname and first name of the patient in question (i.e., Silva, Fulano Souza).

3.6.2 Receiving Data from Another Healthcare Professional

You will receive the compressed data in a file with the patient's surname and first name (i.e., Silva, Fulano Souza). By following the steps described above, identify and open the ResScan™ "Patients" folder. In this folder you must create a folder and rename it with the name of the file you have previously received (in our example, the name of the folder will be "Silva, Fulano Souza"). Unzip the file you received inside this folder (do this with the ResScan™ program closed). Once you open the ResScan™ program, you will see the folder you created in the Patient List. When you open the patient file, all detailed information will be available for your evaluation. But make sure that when you unzip the files the data will be available in the patient root directory (if you unzip this file to a folder inside the patient's folder, you will not be able to view the data when opening the ResScan™ program).

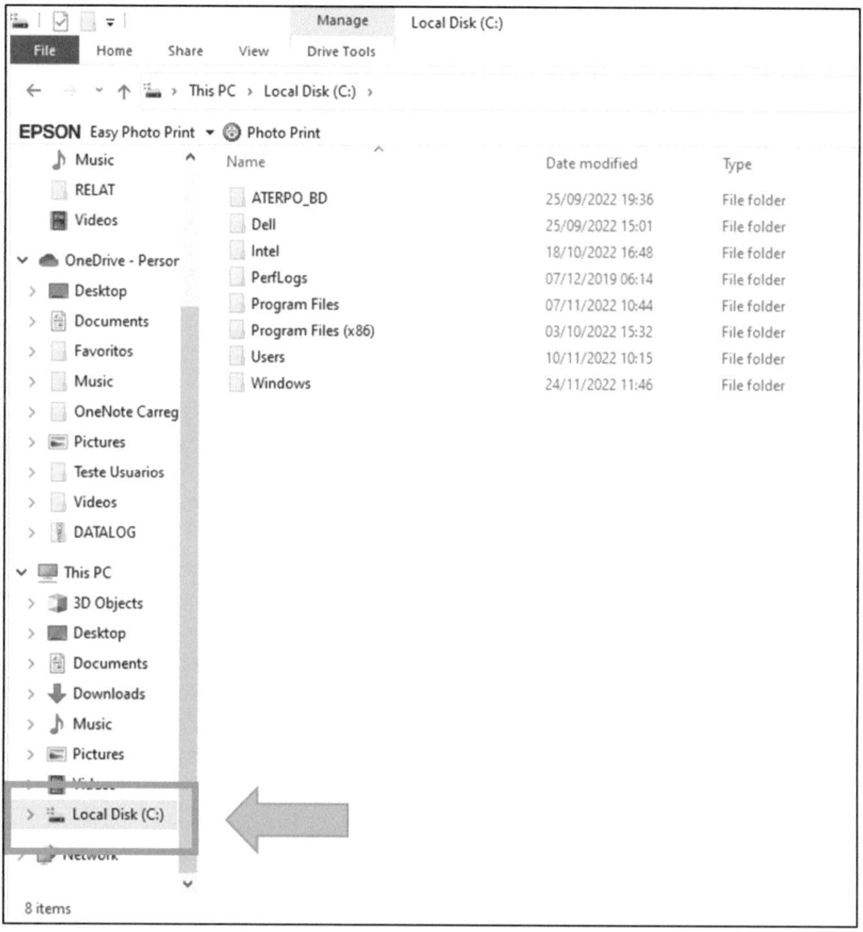

Fig. 3.19 Locating your computer's root folder (arrow). (Figure source: own work)

3.6.3 Instructing the Patient and Receiving the Data

Sometimes the patient needs remote care (e.g., as we saw during the COVID-19 pandemic), and in this case we do not have the SD card on hand. However, advanced graphic information is sometimes crucial for monitoring and adapting therapy in the most challenging cases.

At the same time, many patients are elderly and do not have the computer knowledge to send digital data. So I developed a streamlined protocol to help the patient send me digital data from his PAP devices. I received high-definition digital PAP

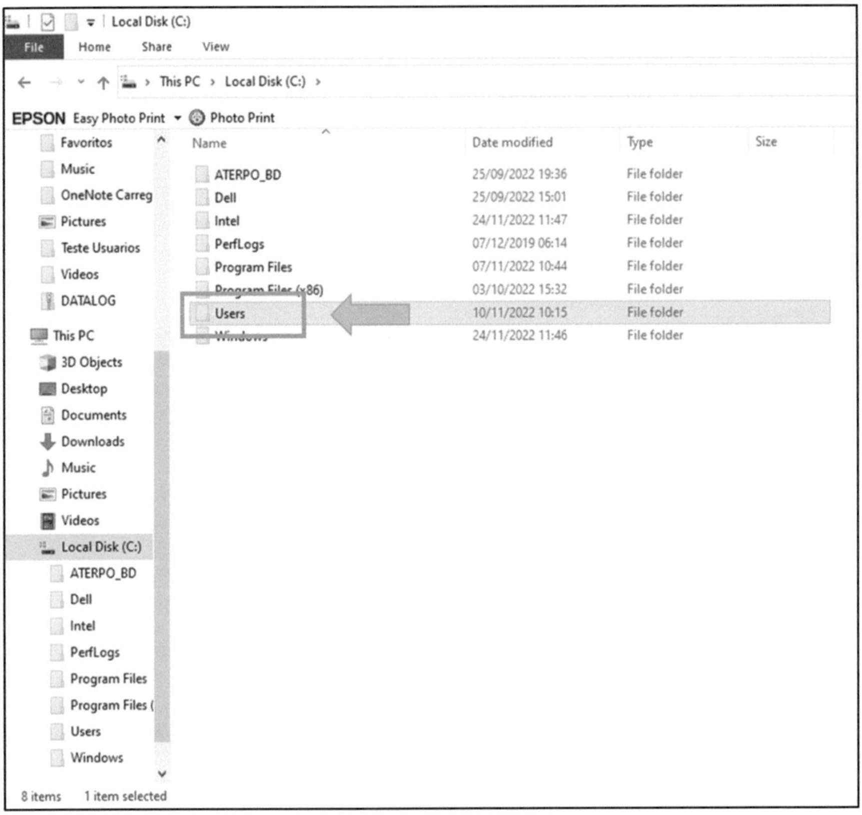

Fig. 3.20 Locating the "Users" folder. (Figure source: own work)

information from my patients in this way, with no major problems. I often guide patients via WhatsApp or videoconference platforms. You will be amazed at how digitally inexperienced patients can use technology when properly instructed. Details of this protocol can be found here.

First, ask the patient to download the PAP SD card onto their own computer. The contents of the card download must appear as shown in Fig. 3.22.

The patient must select all of this content, then right-click the cursor and send it into a "Compressed File". You need to instruct the patient on how to send to you this compressed folder by e-mail (often the content, even if compressed, has been large; in these cases, is better to send it by using GoogleDrive, Dropbox or any other tool that can manage large files) (Fig. 3.23). Inform patients that it is only with the clinical program that this data can be opened (they will not be able to open the data on their PC).

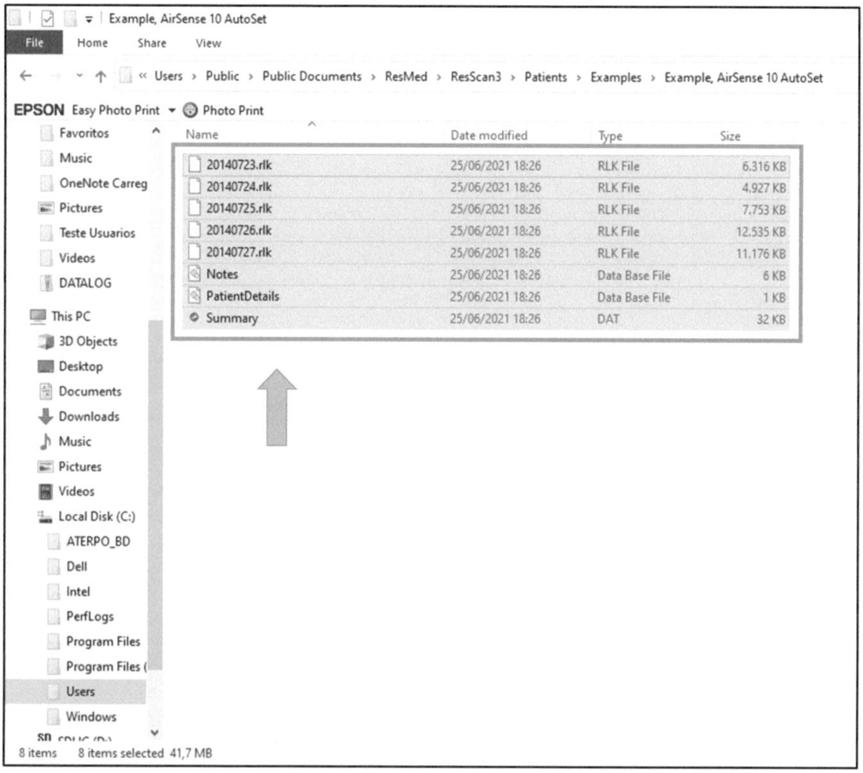

Fig. 3.21 Select all the contents of the "Patient" folder. Right click to select "Send to a compressed file". (Figure source: own work)

When you get this file, you need to copy the contents to an SD card or USB drive. Unzip the file. Check that all the content has been sent to you ("DATALOG" and "SETTINGS" folders, "Identification.tgt", "Identification.crc", and "STR.edf" files). If the files come in under different names, they will not be recognized by the ResScan™ system. If this is the case, rename the files to properly manage archives (Fig. 3.24).

As previously advised, inside the SD card or on the pen drive, the data card file may not be in the subfolders, it should be just below the root directory. When you unzip the file, a subdirectory is generally created. Select all the contents of the subfolder and paste directly under the root folder of the SD card or pen drive. Now just open ResScan™ and the program will recognize the contents of your SD card or USB stick as if it were the card of the patient's device. As a tip, you can do so with any device of any manufacturer.

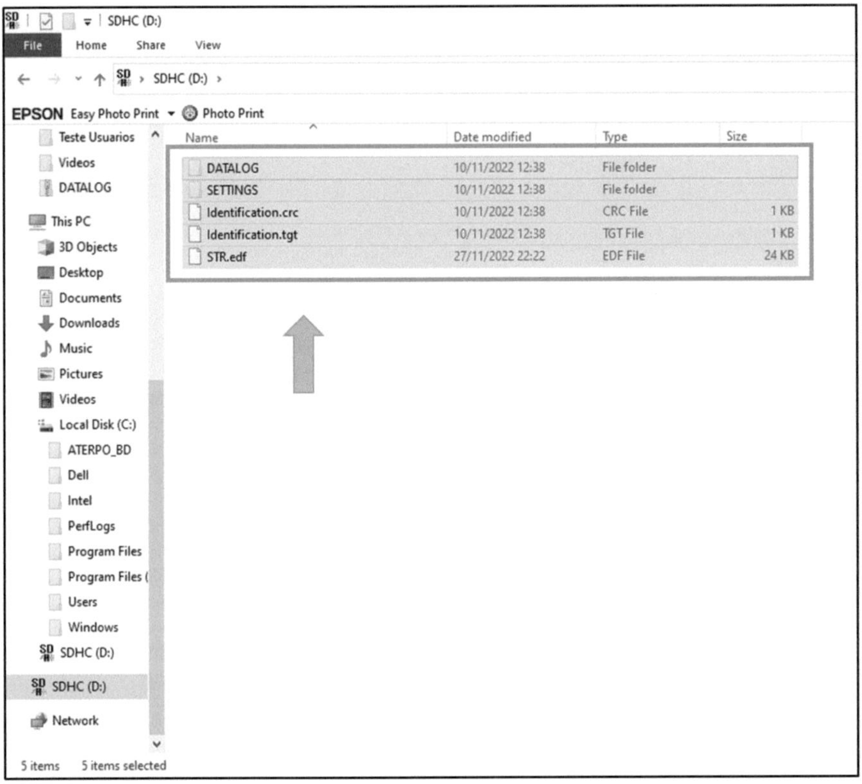

Fig. 3.22 When the patient downloads the data onto their own computer, the contents of the SD card are presented in this way (arrow). (Figure source: own work)

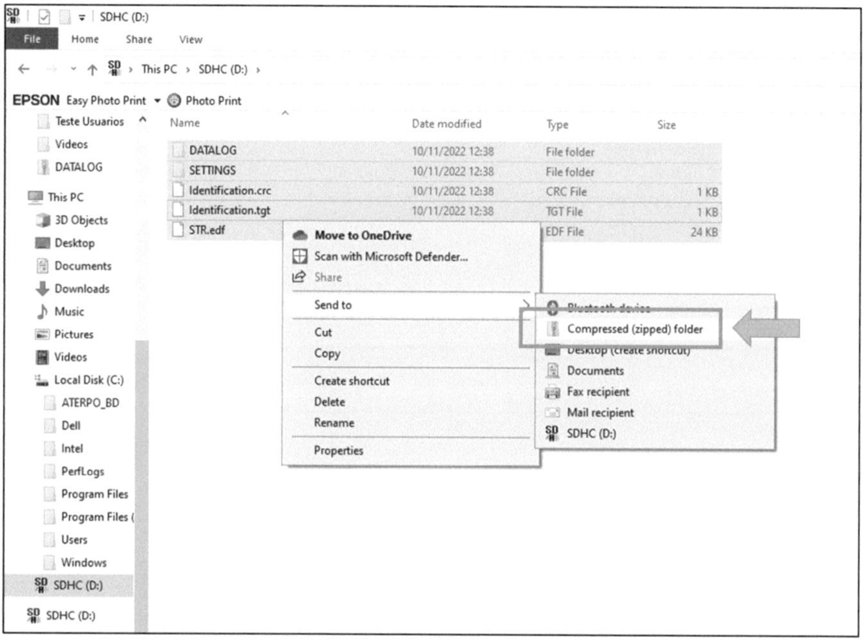

Fig. 3.23 The patient must select all folder content, then right click the cursor, and send it to a "Compressed File". You need to instruct the patient on how to send to you this compressed folder by e-mail (often the content, even if compressed, has been large; in these cases, is better to send it by using GoogleDrive, Dropbox, or any other tool that can manage large files). (Figure source: own work)

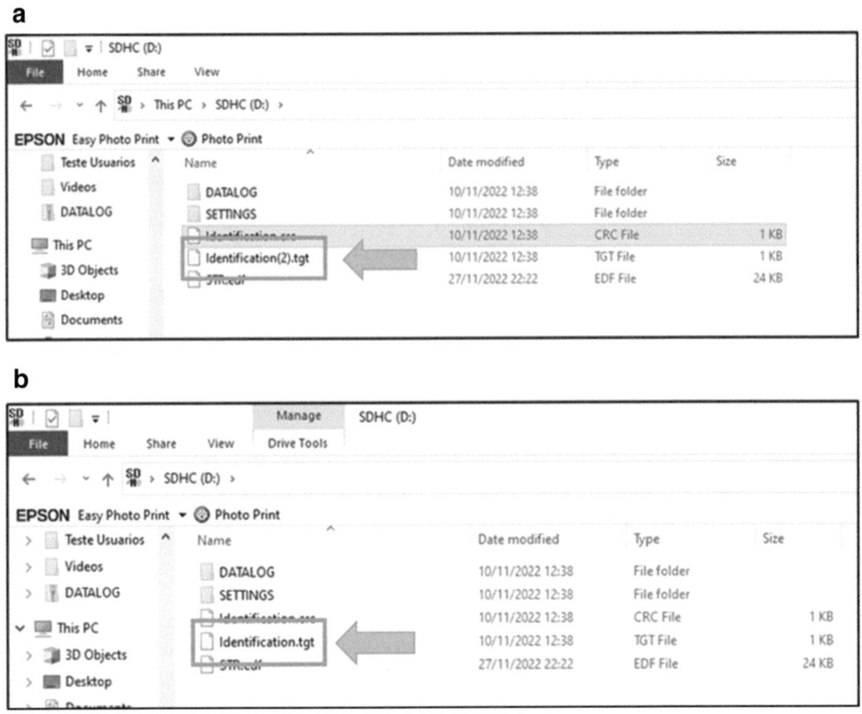

Fig. 3.24 In this example, the data file came with the name “Identification(2).tgt” and was renamed to “Identification.tgt” to be properly recognized by the ResScan™ system. (Figure source: own work)

3.7 Procedure when Respiratory Flow Curve Is Not Displayed

Ensure to have the latest version of the ResScan™ software. Be careful to always work with the latest software for any positive pressure equipment manufacturer you want to analyze high-resolution data.

Install a new version, if applicable. However, if this does not resolve the problem, follow these steps.

3.7.1 First Options for Showing the Flow Curve

On the ResScan™ home screen, click on the “Reports” option (Fig. 3.25). Then click on the “Customize” option (Fig. 3.26). Click on the “Detailed Graphs” option (Fig. 3.27). Confirm that the “Flow” plots are in this window. Otherwise, add the

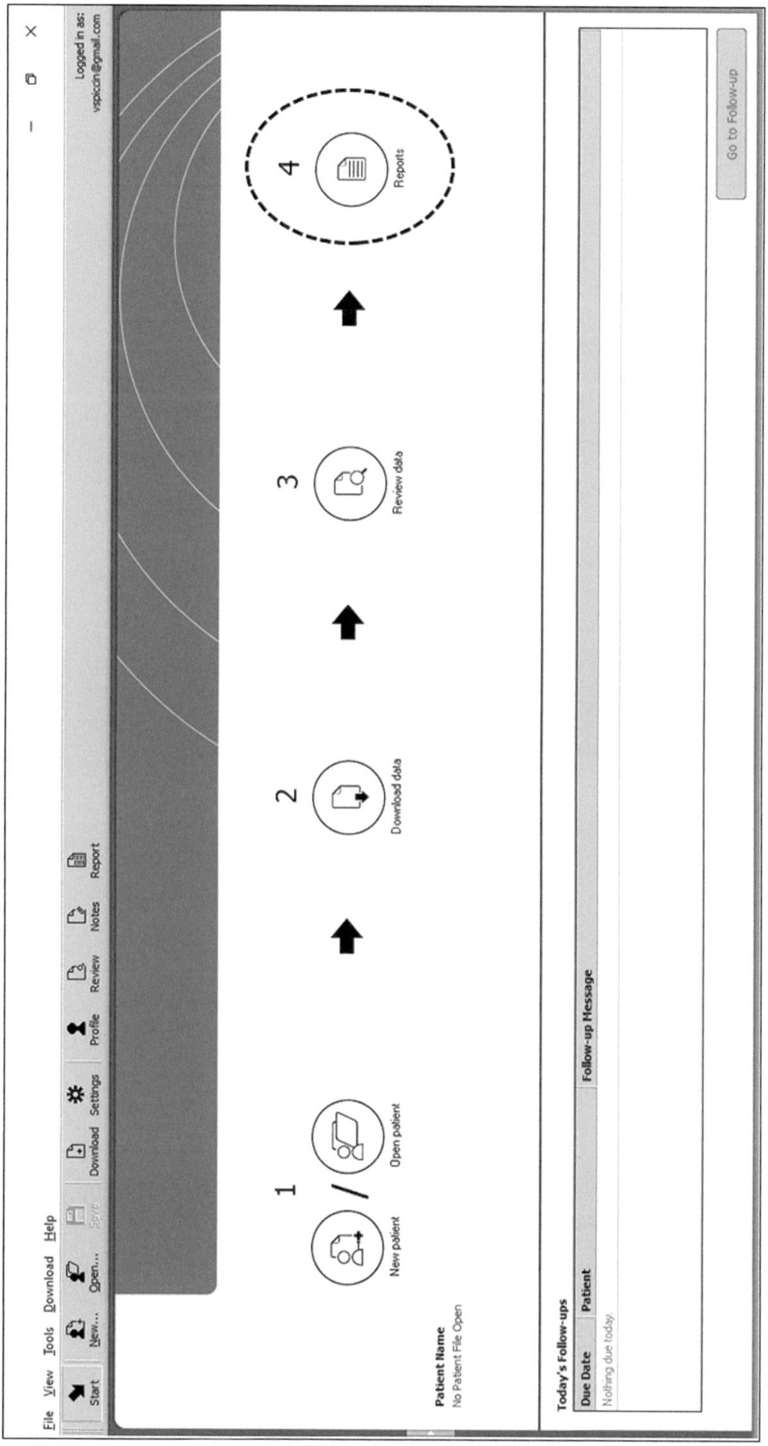

Fig. 3.25 Click on the "Reports" option. (Figure Copyright ResMed (with permission))

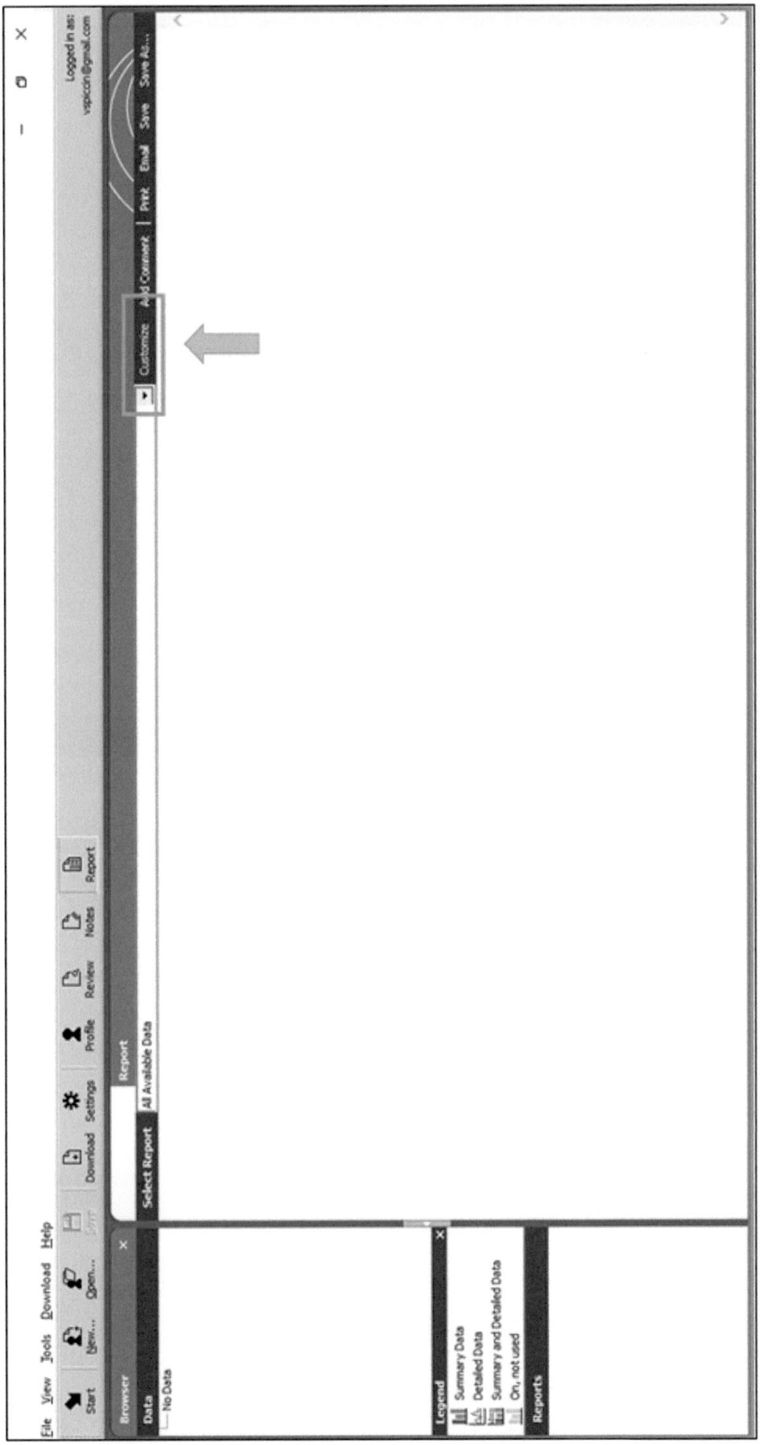

Fig. 3.26 Click the Customize option. (Figure Copyright ResMed (with permission))

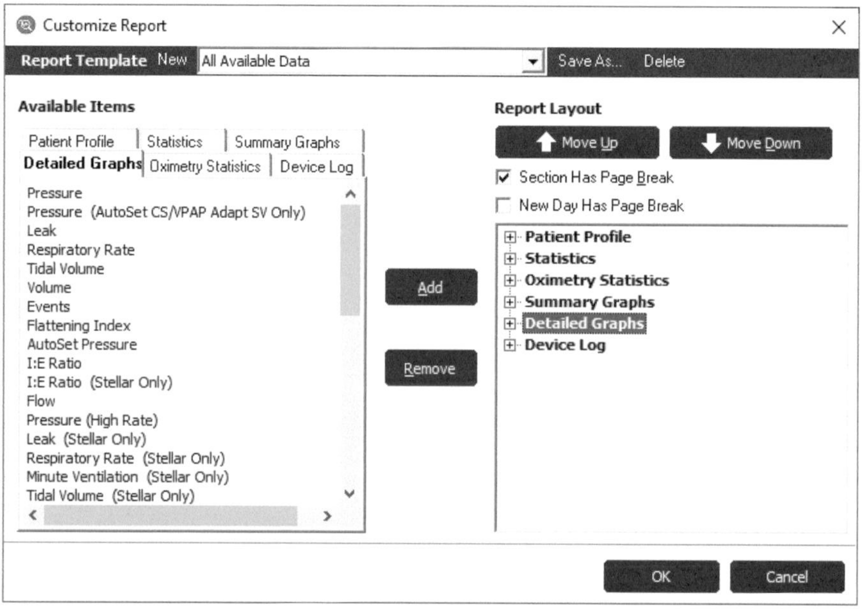

Fig. 3.27 Click in the window on the right, on the Detailed Graph option. (Figure Copyright ResMed (with permission))

"Flow" plots in this window. If it is not, look for the "Flow" option in the left window, select this option and clicking the ADD button between the two windows (Fig. 3.28).

3.7.2 *Second Option for Viewing the Flow Curve*

Check on the "Navigation" screen that the "Flow" is correctly selected and that the number of visible graphs corresponds to the option selected (Fig. 3.29).

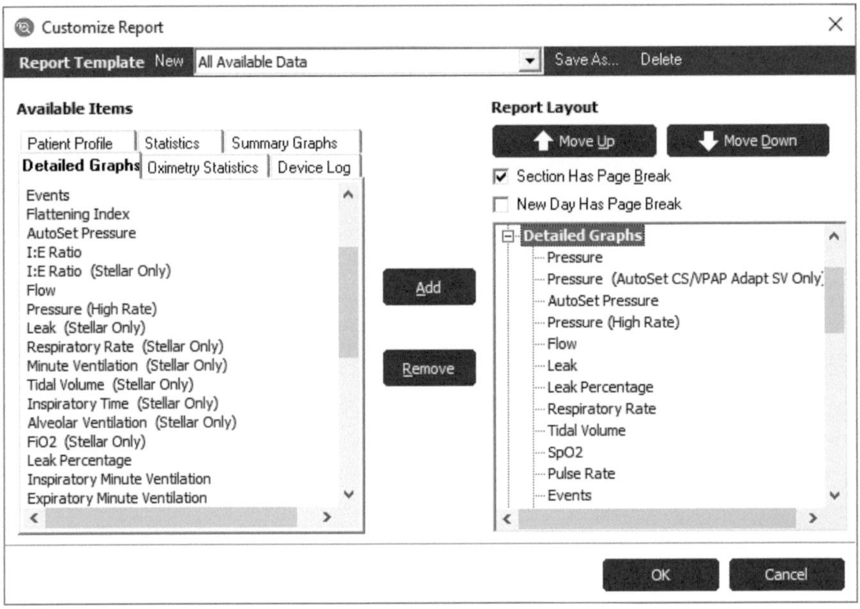

Fig. 3.28 Confirm that the "Flow" plot is in the Detailed Graphs window. Otherwise, add the Flow plot in this window looking for the "Flow" option in the left window, select this option, and click the ADD button between the two windows. (Figure Copyright ResMed (with permission))

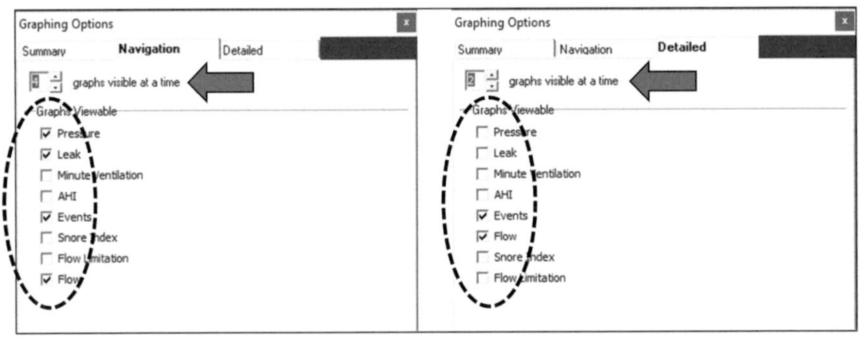

Fig. 3.29 Check that the "Flow" is properly selected on the "Navigation" screen (dotted circle) and that the number of visible graphs matches the option you selected (arrow). (Figure Copyright ResMed (with permission))

3.8 Further Reading

Airflow analysis is also discussed in the book Advances in the Diagnosis and Treatment of Sleep Apnea (series title: Advances in Experimental Medicine and Biology—doi.org/10.1007/978-3-031-06413-5). The chapter "Airflow Analysis in the Context of Sleep Apnea" reviews the main methodological approaches applied to characterize and extract relevant information from respiratory airflow signal [12].

References

1. Gay P, Weaver T, Loube D, Iber C, Force PAPT, SoP C, et al. Evaluation of positive airway pressure treatment for sleep related breathing disorders in adults. Sleep. 2006;29(3):381–401.
2. Weaver TE, Maislin G, Dinges DF, Bloxham T, George CF, Greenberg H, et al. Relationship between hours of CPAP use and achieving normal levels of sleepiness and daily functioning. Sleep. 2007;30(6):711–9. https://doi.org/10.1093/sleep/30.6.711.
3. Guerrero A, Embid C, Farre R, Navajas D, Masa JF, Duran J, et al. Sleep breathing flow characteristics as a sign for the detection of wakefulness in patients with sleep apnea. Respiration. 2010;80(6):495–9. https://doi.org/10.1159/000264656.
4. Ayappa I, Norman RG, Whiting D, Tsai AH, Anderson F, Donnely E, et al. Irregular respiration as a marker of wakefulness during titration of CPAP. Sleep. 2009;32(1):99–104.
5. Ayappa I, Norman RG, Suryadevara M, Rapoport DM. Comparison of limited monitoring using a nasal-cannula flow signal to full polysomnography in sleep-disordered breathing. Sleep. 2004;27(6):1171–9. https://doi.org/10.1093/sleep/27.6.1171.
6. Hosselet JJ, Norman RG, Ayappa I, Rapoport DM. Detection of flow limitation with a nasal cannula/pressure transducer system. Am J Respir Crit Care Med. 1998;157(5 Pt 1):1461–7.
7. Nguyen CD, Amatoury J, Carberry JC, Eckert DJ. An automated and reliable method for breath detection during variable mask pressures in awake and sleeping humans. PLoS One. 2017;12(6):e0179030. https://doi.org/10.1371/journal.pone.0179030.
8. Al-Halhouli A, Al-Ghussain L, El Bouri S, Liu H, Zheng D. Clinical evaluation of stretchable and wearable inkjet-printed strain gauge sensor for respiratory rate monitoring at different measurements locations. J Clin Monit Comput. 2021;35(3):453–62. https://doi.org/10.1007/s10877-020-00481-3.
9. Arora N, Meskill G, Guilleminault C. The role of flow limitation as an important diagnostic tool and clinical finding in mild sleep-disordered breathing. Sleep Sci. 2015;8(3):134–42. https://doi.org/10.1016/j.slsci.2015.08.003.
10. Rapoport D, Norman R, Nielson M. Nasal pressure airflow measurement–an introduction. Corpus Christi, TX: Pro-Tech. Services; 2001.
11. Berry RB, Brooks R, Gamaldo C, Harding SM, Lloyd RM, Quan SF, et al. AASM scoring manual updates for 2017 (version 2.4). J Clin Sleep Med. 2017;13(5):665–6. https://doi.org/10.5664/jcsm.6576.
12. Barroso-García V, Jiménez-García J, Gutiérrez-Tobal GC, Hornero R. Airflow analysis in the context of sleep apnea. In: Penzel T, Hornero R, editors. Advances in the diagnosis and treatment of sleep apnea: filling the gap between physicians and engineers. Cham: Springer; 2022. p. 241–53.

Chapter 4
Assessment of the Respiratory Flow Curve

4.1 Understanding of Algorithms

Polysomnography (PSG) is a sleep study that uses electroencephalogram, electro-oculogram, electromyogram, electrocardiogram, and pulse oximetry, as well as airflow and respiratory effort, to assess the underlying causes of sleep disturbance. Two quality airflow sensors are used in the PSG. The oronasal thermal sensor (thermistor) detects temperature changes in inhaled or exhaled respiration to monitor airflow and is best used to identify apneas (90% reduction in airflow). The nasal pressure transducer detects pressure changes during inhalation and exhalation to monitor airflow and is used to identify hypopnea (30% reduction of airflow). In addition, two respiratory inductance plethysmography sensors or straps are used to determine the qualitative respiratory effort in the chest and abdomen. These sensors identify the various types of respiratory events, including obstructive apnea, obstructive hypopnea, and central apnea [1].

During the PSG examination, oxygen saturation is obtained through pulse oximetry and is used to assist with scoring hypopneas when there is at least a 3% or 4% oxygen desaturation (depending on whether the recommended AASM or acceptable scoring criteria is used) associated with the respiratory event. Also, PSG detects arousals from sleep stages N1, N2, N3, or REM when there is an abrupt shift of the electroencephalogram frequency in the alpha or theta range, or frequencies greater than 16 Hz, lasting for at least 3 s [1].

PSG is the gold standard for diagnosing sleep-related breathing disorders, which include obstructive sleep apnea (OSA), central sleep apnea, and sleep-related hypoventilation/hypoxia [1].

Positive airway pressure (PAP) devices – like continuous, auto-adjusting, and bilevel machines, can also measure airflow and circuit pressure to detect and store the memory mask on time and the occurrence of respiratory events. The algorithms

V. S. Piccin, *Monitoring Positive Pressure Therapy in Sleep-Related Breathing Disorders*, https://doi.org/10.1007/978-3-031-50292-7_4

for event detection used by these devices are based on measurements of airflow, vibration, and airflow profile flattening [2].

Detection of events from PAP devices shows the same variables obtained on polysomnogram (PSG), including apnea-hypopnea index (AHI), apnea index (AI), and hypopnea index (HI). However, although health professionals use the event detection information recorded by these PAP devices to assess treatment efficacy, PAP devices and PSG differ in the methods used to generate these measures. PAPs use airflow to detect apnea and hypopnea. In contrast, the abnormal respiratory events on PSG are scored using not only airflow but also the arterial oxygen saturation level, respiratory effort, and, depending on the scoring criteria, electroencephalographic (EEG)/electromyographic (EMG) arousals.

Due to differences in how PAP and PSG detect respiratory events and generate indices of respiratory events, it is very important that healthcare practitioners understand how these measures compare to each other [2].

It is also essential for sleep care professionals to be aware that each manufacturer has developed their own algorithm for their positive airway pressure machines. In this book, we discuss the algorithm developed for ResMed for devices commonly used to treat sleep apnea.

4.1.1 *Obstructive or Central Apneas*

When analyzing the respiratory flow curve generated by the PAP device, in regular respiration, the respiratory flow curve will have a characteristic design, as shown in Fig. 4.1.

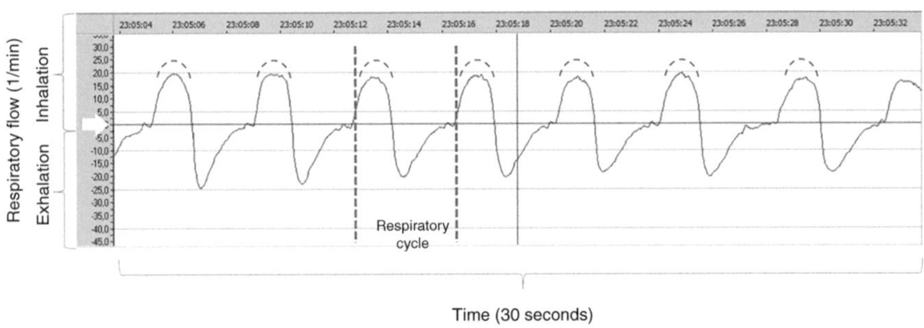

Fig. 4.1 The arrow shows the "zero"point which marks the transition from inspiration to exhalation. We note here that the inhalation curve is relatively rounded (half circle dashed), and that the expiration curve is slightly longer than the inhalation curve. Inhalation ends at the beginning of exhaling and exhaling ends at the beginning of inhalation. The sum of an inspiratory curve and an exhalation curve is referred to as the breathing cycle and appears as a sine wave (dashed parallel bars). In a one-minute window, we should expect to find 14–20 breathing cycles (here we have a 30-s window to better observe the respiratory waveform). In general, we expect the maximum inspiratory flow rate to be about 20 L/min, but this value will show some individual variations. (Source: author's collection)

The device analyzes the condition of the patient's upper airway for each breath and delivers pressure within the allowed range depending on the degree of obstruction. When the patient is breathing normally, the inspiratory flow measured by the device as a function of time shows a typically rounded curve for each breath, as shown in Fig. 4.1. The algorithm recognizes apnea through the temporary absence or disruption of the respiratory flow curve. Apnea is recorded when there is a 75% decrease in respiration from baseline for at least 10 s. ResScan™ shows three types of apneas: central apnea (apnea during which the airway remains open), obstructive apnea (apnea during which there is physical closure of the upper airway), and unknown apnea (apnea during which there is leakage greater than 30 L/min, which prevents the exact determination of the type of apnea—obstructive or central) (Fig. 4.2).

To define if there is an obstructive or central respiratory event, after a 4 s lack of the respiratory flow the ResMed algorithm triggers a vibrating wave for another 6 s (forced oscillation technique, which applies small oscillations of 4 Hz to the pressure generated by the device). The return of this wave (represented by changes in the flow signal, that is, the vibratory wave "found" a mechanical resistance) indicates a mechanical obstruction of the upper airway (UA) that, adding to the 10 s respiratory flow lack interval, will result in the recording of an obstructive apnea. Under the same conditions, but without return of the vibratory wave signal (i.e., without changes in the flow signal – which means that the signal generated by the vibratory wave did not "find" resistance in its passage), indicates an apnea without the obstruction of the UA, and the device will register a central apnea (Fig. 4.3). Figure 4.4 displays the forced oscillation signal on the respiratory flow curve.

When an automatic device is used, there are some different responses to each specific respiratory event. In an obstructive apnea, the algorithm increases pressure to keep the airway open and prevent further obstructive events. When a central apnea occurs, the machine does not increase pressure (increasing pressure for central respiratory events may cause discomfort to the patient). Mixed apneas are usually classified as obstructive apneas and, in these respiratory events the PAP pressure increases. If the leak is too high or the device cannot determine the type of apnea, it

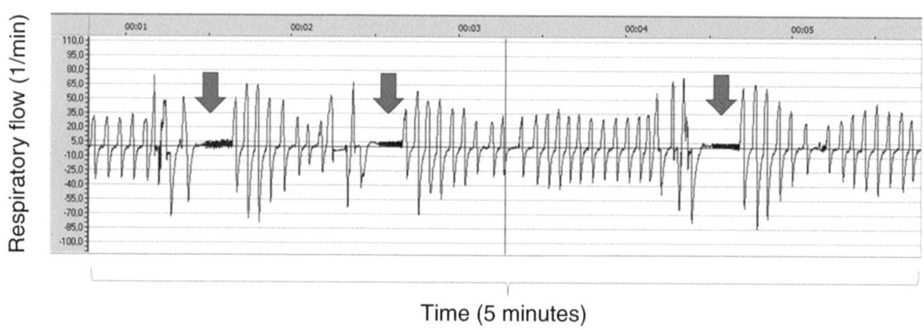

Fig. 4.2 Apnea is a lack of breathing flow over a period of more than 10 s (arrow). In the Y axis, the respiratory flow rate is expressed in liters per minute. (Source: author's collection)

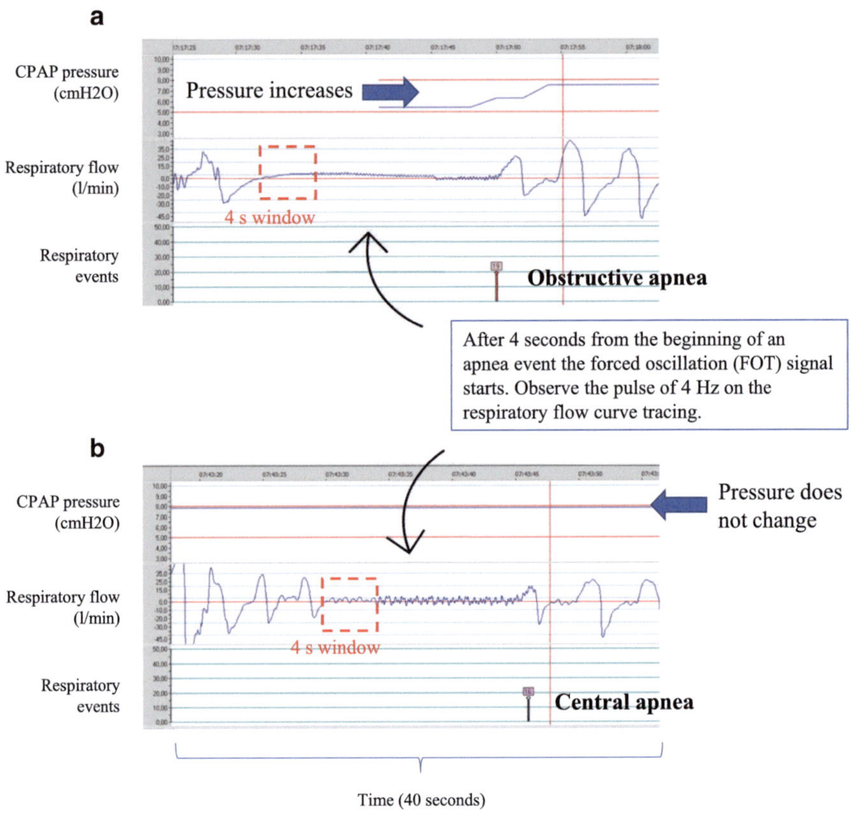

Fig. 4.3 It is a representation of the ResMed positive airway pressure algorithm for detecting respiratory events (for sleep apnea treatment devices). After 4 s of apnea onset, a 4 Hz oscillatory frequency (FOT) signal is initiated. If there is a return of the forced oscillation signal (**a**), the upper airway is closed (the device understands that there is an obstructive apnea, and CPAP pressure increases); if the forced oscillation signal does not return (**b**), the upper airway is open (in this case, the event is distinguished as a central apnea and the CPAP pressure does not change). (Source: author's collection)

is classified as an unknown apnea (and in face of this event, the PAP algorithm does not increase the positive airway pressure).

4.1.2 Mixed Apnea

Mixed apnea is a combination of central apnea events and obstructive apnea events. Because the device cannot tell whether there is a chest wall motion, it cannot rule out the possibility of closed central apneas (mixed apneas). It only sees that the

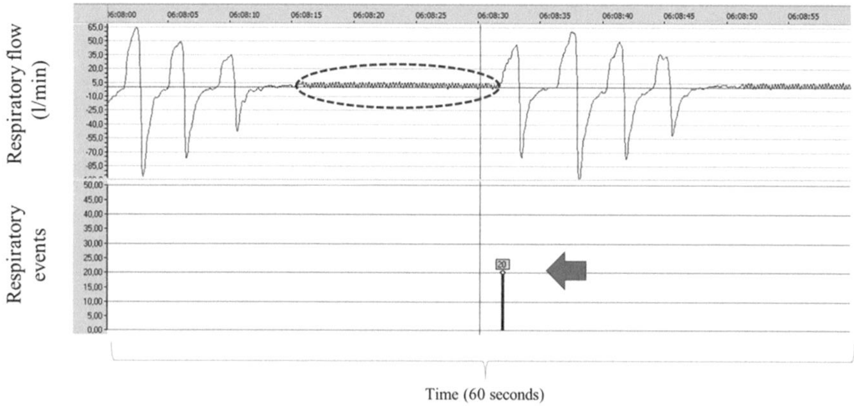

Fig. 4.4 Serrated line (dashed circle) resulting from the application of the forced oscillation technique to distinguish central/obstructive apneas. The Y axis shows the respiratory events and respiratory flow. In this example, using the forced oscillation technique, the device algorithm identified a central apnea event (arrow), with a duration of 20 s. (Source: author's collection)

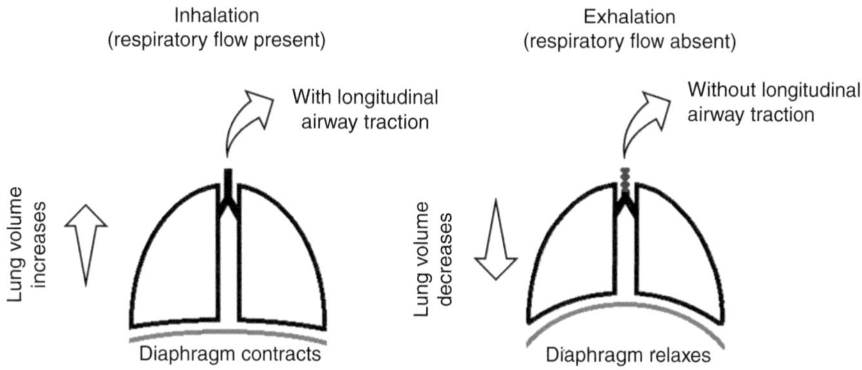

Fig. 4.5 In case of inspiration, the pulmonary volume keeps the upper airway (UA) stabilized; in the absence of inspiratory flow, the UA loses its stability and tends to collapse. Modified after ©Movements of the diaphragm and lungs during inspiration by sportEX journals under CC BY-ND 2.0

airway is closed and treats these events like obstructive apnea. Thus, generally mixed apneas are categorized as obstructive respiratory events by the PAP algorithm.

Nowadays some authors consider that mixed apnea can be treated as a central event [3]. We must bear in mind that in mixed apnea, the very cessation of respiratory flow, due to central apnea, destabilizes and prevents the maintenance of airway permeability, culminating in the closure of the upper airways [4, 5]. Many researchers believe that the upper airway obstruction occurs as a consequence of the lung volume decrease with the breathing cessation (so, an UA obstruction takes place because of the loss of the tracheal traction) (Fig. 4.5) [6, 7].

The knowledge of the behavior of the respiratory flow as well as the shape of the respiratory flow curve allows assessment of when there is a mixed apnea event (which allows us, many times, to be more accurate with the therapeutic strategies adopted). However, mixed apnea is not an easy phenomenon to detect and requires a good technical knowledge of the characteristics of breathing patterns during sleep (Fig. 4.6). In addition, knowledge of a patient's clinical history is important in defining these events.

4.1.3 *Obstructive or Central Hypopnea*

Regarding hypopnea events, we must first remember that the American Academy of Sleep Medicine (AASM), recommended to score a respiratory event as a hypopnea if all of the following criteria are met: the peak signal excursions drop by ≥30% of pre-event baseline using nasal pressure (diagnostic study), PAP device flow (titration study), or an alternative hypopnea sensor (diagnostic study); the duration of the ≥30% drop in signal excursion is ≥10 s; there is a ≥ 3% oxygen desaturation from pre-event baseline and/or the event is associated with an arousal. Also is acceptable to score a respiratory event as a hypopnea if all of the following criteria are met: the

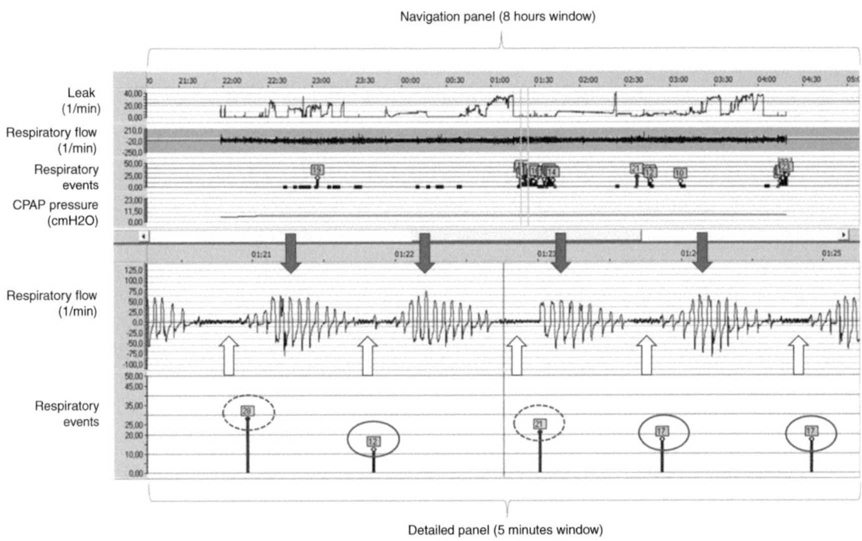

Fig. 4.6 Note in this example that the same respiratory flow pattern (hyperventilation – closed arrows, and apnea – open arrows) is sometimes characterized by the algorithm as a central respiratory event (closed circle) and other times as an obstructive event (dotted circle). Probably the very cessation of the respiratory flow destabilizes the permeability of the upper airways, resulting in the closure of the upper airways. The statistical report will check for many obstructive residual events that should be considered as residual central apnea events. Visualizing the respiratory flow curve during sleep allows us to better direct therapy. (Source: author's collection)

peak signal excursions drop by ≥30% of pre-event baseline using nasal pressure (diagnostic study), PAP device flow (titration study), or an alternative hypopnea sensor (diagnostic study); the duration of the ≥30% drop in signal excursion is ≥10 s; there is a ≥ 4% oxygen desaturation from pre-event baseline (note that the criterion involving arousals is included only in the recommended criteria to score an hypopnea event, and excluded from acceptable criteria) [8, 9].

Hypopneas can be caused by the partial obstruction of the airway, which causes a sequence of flow-limited inspirations (obstructive in origin), or shallow breathing, which is not associated with any flow limitation (central in origin).

The PAP algorithm determines that hypopnea events occur by identifying the decrease in the amplitude of the breathing flow curve. The enhanced ResMed algorithm identifies hypopnea as a reduction in airflow of 50% or more for 10 s or more (Fig. 4.7). For the device to qualify an event as a hypopnea, it must meet all these criteria: the flow limitation is at least 10 s long, there is a flow limited breath, and the respiratory event is not part of an (eventual) apnea. The flow limitation should be preceded by normal breathing which can be used as a parameter for calculating reduced respiratory flow.

The monitoring of hypopnea events by the ResMed PAP algorithm is very close to what is recommended by the AASM guidelines. However, we must remember that since the device does not measure blood oxygen saturation or arousal, the hypopnea index provided is not completely reliable according to AASM guidelines. This does not mean that the algorithms are not good enough, but that we need to understand the limits that exist to better interpret the results.

To distinguish between obstructive and central hypopnea events, it is very important to pay close attention to the morphology of the inspiratory flow curve. Characteristically, central hypopneas show no flattening of the inspiratory flow curve and obstructive hypopneas show this flattening (due to upper airway obstruction, as shown in Fig. 4.8). However, we cannot exclude the possibility that a small reduction in inspiratory amplitude, by the reduced drive, leads to the loss of UA support, causing an obstructive hypopnea in the course of an initial central hypopnea [10, 11].

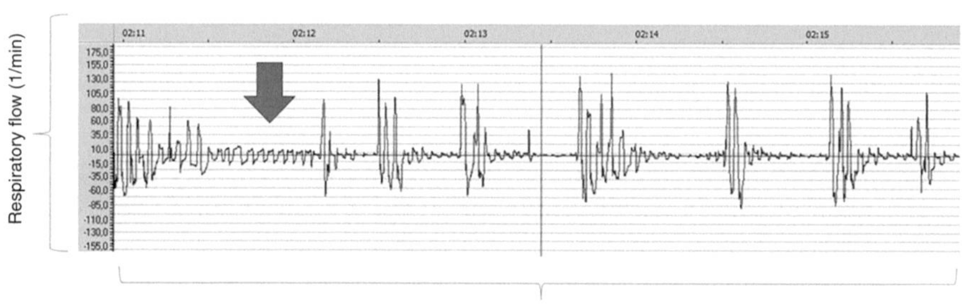

Fig. 4.7 Examples of hypopnea breathing (arrow), where there is up to 50% reduction in breathing (compared to baseline) associated with partial airway obstruction for at least 10 s. On the Y axis, the respiratory flow rate is in liters per minute. (Source: author's collection)

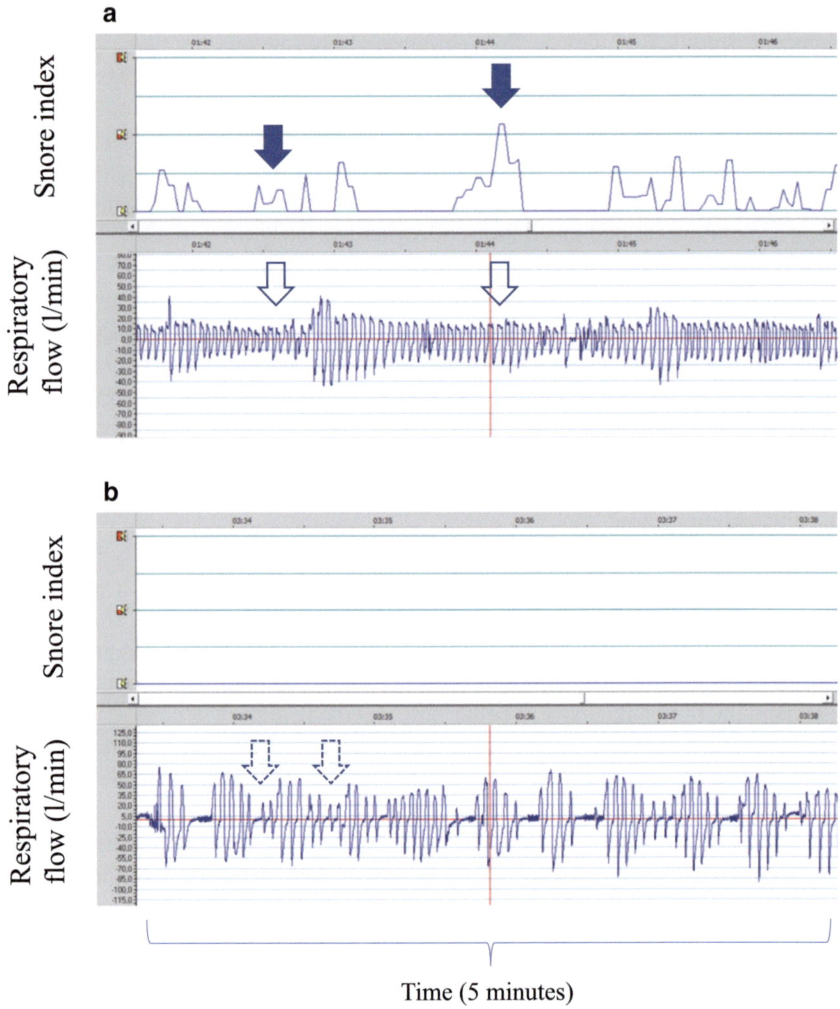

Fig. 4.8 (**a**) Note the characteristic of the respiratory flow showing a flattening of the inspiratory flow (open arrow). The flow restriction also has a snoring signal (filled arrow). (**b**) The inspiratory flow is reduced, but the inspiratory flow curve is not flattened (dashed arrow). There is no snoring on (**b**). (Source: author's collection)

When obstructive hypopnea occurs, inspiratory flattening can take several forms (Fig. 4.9).

Recently, some studies related the morphology of flow curves in an event of obstructive hypopnea, with specific anatomical alterations of the UA [13–16]. For example, the shape of the inspiratory flow curve in an obstructive hypopnea event could indicate an isolated palatal and lateral collapse compared to individuals with characteristics of greater obstruction posteriorly at the base of the tongue (Fig. 4.10).

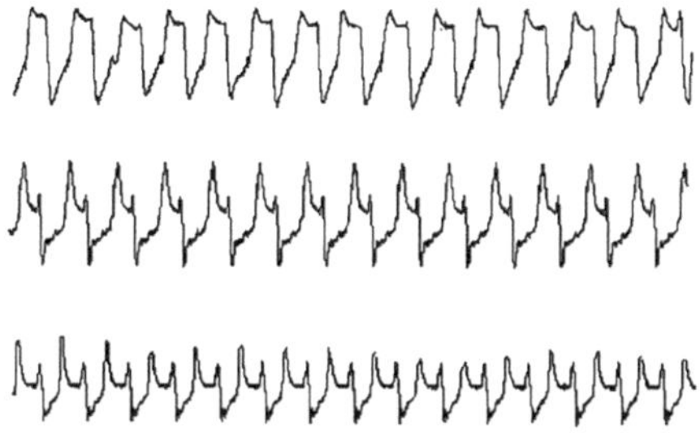

Fig. 4.9 In this figure observe three examples of obstructive hypopneas, showing variations on the inspiratory flow pattern (flat: 1/M-shapes: 2 and 3). The flow limitation is due to an upper airway collapse resulting from an imbalance between high negative esophageal pressure and low upper airway muscle activity. In this figure inspiration corresponds to upward flow. (Source: Calero et al., 2006 (with permission) [12])

On the other hand, the format of the exhalation flow curve could also explain the mechanism of mouth air leaking through palatal prolapse (Fig. 4.11) [15, 17].

The relation between the flow curve and the anatomy of the UA could facilitate treatments targeting specific subgroups of individuals. It is interesting to note that the ResMed algorithm measures inspiratory flow limitation by measuring the shape of the inspiratory flow-time curve (3-breath moving average). This prevents automatic devices from reacting to random respiratory events, such as sighing or coughing, while providing a breath-to-breath response. AutoSet™ devices provide a pressure response to flow limitation by evaluating the shape of the curve under tidal volume (compared to recent ventilation) and the elongation of the flow curve, called time of inspiratory (TI) stretching, which may indicate that the patient is expending more energy to breathe. Also, AutoSet™ responds to respiratory flow curve limitations, even if these curves have an unusual shape (known as M-shapes), as seen in Fig. 4.9. But the AutoSet™ response does not treat atypical M-shaped breath without TI stretching or drop in tidal volume, as it can be caused by artifacts of the cardiogenic flow on the respiratory flow curve (Fig. 4.12).

4.1.4 *Respiratory Effort-Related Arousal*

Obstructive events can be considered as a continuum of partial to complete blockage of the upper airways. Upper airway resistance occurs early in this spectrum and describes events where upper airway resistance increases during sleep and is detected as a restriction of flow during polysomnography, without hypopnea parameters. This increase in upper airway resistance could increase breathing work, causing arousals and disrupted sleep [18]. That respiratory phenomenon, usually called as respiratory effort-related arousals (RERA), are characterized by respiratory events without concomitant oxygen desaturation, which may lead to daytime sleepiness and functional impairment. Several previous studies have attempted to

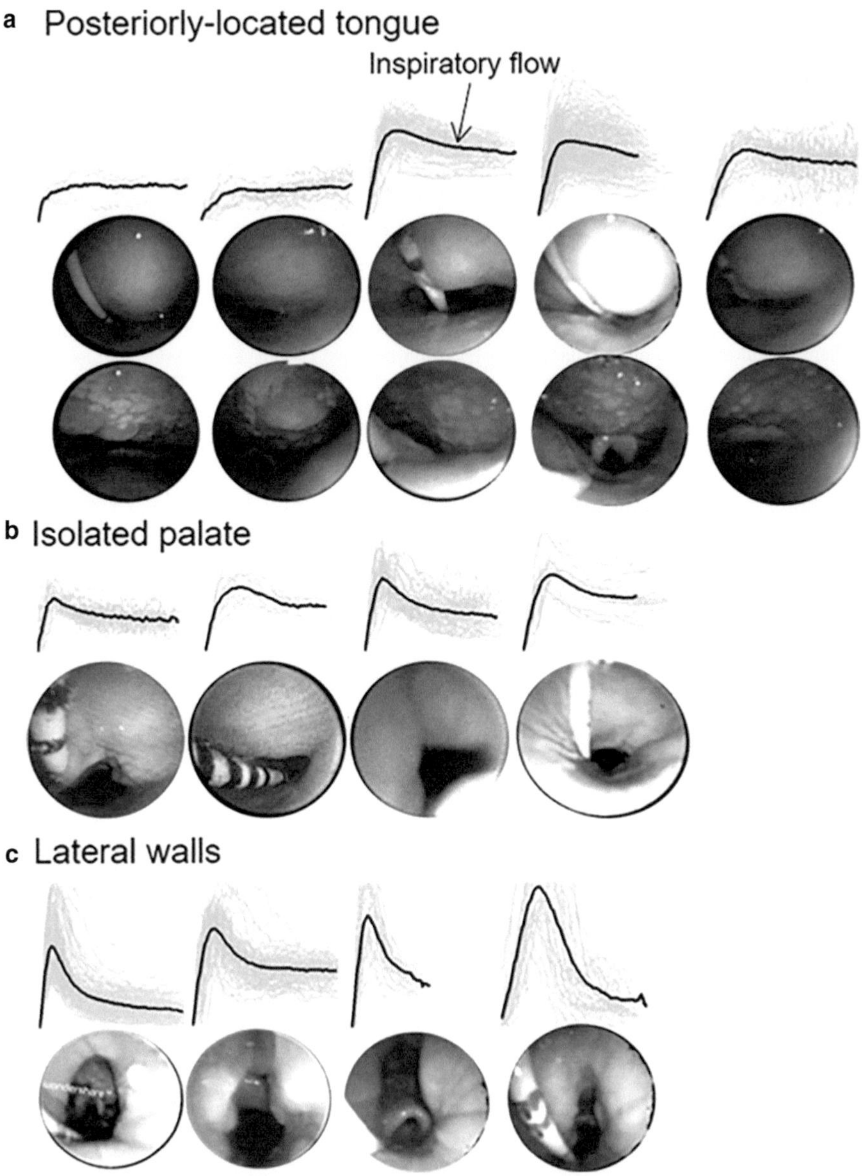

Fig. 4.10 Representative examples of various inspirational flow patterns. The darkest lines over the images represent the average inspiratory flow of the set of inspiratory flow plots. Note that the inspiratory flow is more spiculated (in other words, it is more dependent on negative effort) among individuals with isolated palatal and lateral collapse compared to individuals with characteristics of greater obstruction posteriorly at the base of the tongue. (**a**) Soft palate, (**b**) Lateral walls, and (**c**) Base of the tongue. (Modified after Genta et al., 2017 (with permission) [13])

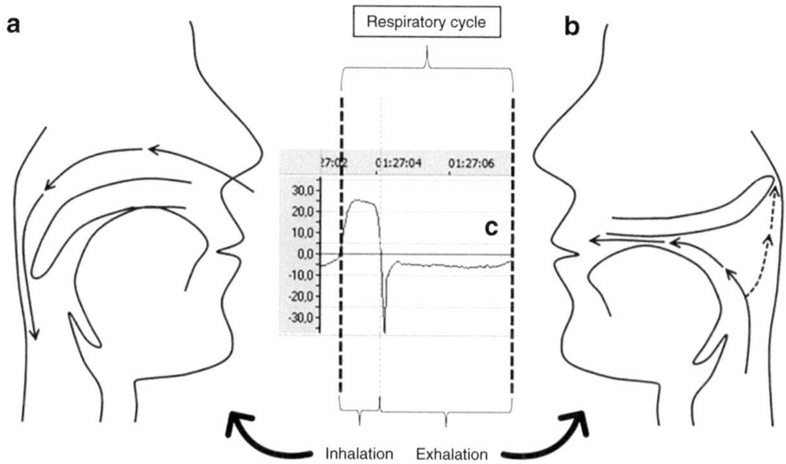

Fig. 4.11 Different oral airflow mechanisms during continuous positive airway nasal pressure (CPAP). (**a**) Normal nasal inspiration: note that the tongue is coupled at the palate; (**b**) Expiratory buccal leak: the palatal prolapse blocks the nasopharynx and the air leaks through the mouth; note that the mouth is open and there is no coupling between the palate and the tongue. In image C observe the airflow characteristic in the inspiratory phase (normal) of the respiratory cycle, and the change in the exhalation phase, where the flow curve is "amputated" (this would be the sign of palatal prolapse while using the CPAP). Image C shows the respiration flow curve in the breathing cycle (l/min). (Modified after Azarbarzin et al., 2018 (with permission) [15])

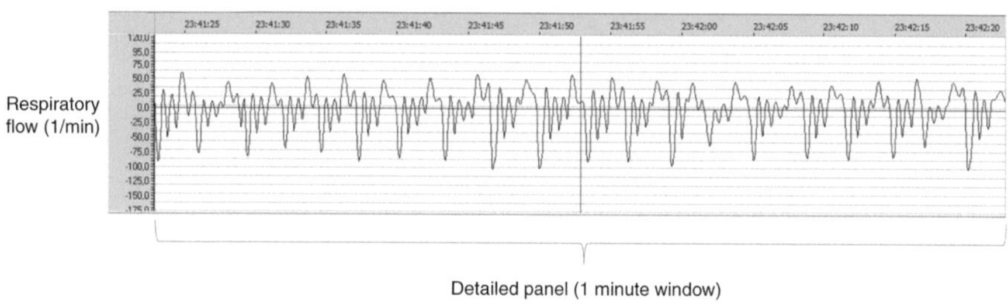

Fig. 4.12 Examples of atypical morphology of the respiratory flow curve, without extending the flow curve or decreasing the current volume. This form of atypical flow may be caused by cardiac flow artifacts on the respiratory flow curve. In this figure inspiration corresponds to upward flow. (Source: own work)

characterize RERA, but their relevance as a specific disorder and their cardiovascular consequences are still a matter of debate [19].

At RERA, the respiratory flow is limited regardless of the effort generated by the respiratory muscles to restore their normal range, and this effort often results in an arousal to restore the breathing pattern even before there is a significant gasometrical change. The gold standard for diagnosing RERA is to apply an esophageal balloon, which will measure respiratory efforts suggesting an increased respiratory effort (Fig. 4.13). This technique, however, is invasive and is not commonly

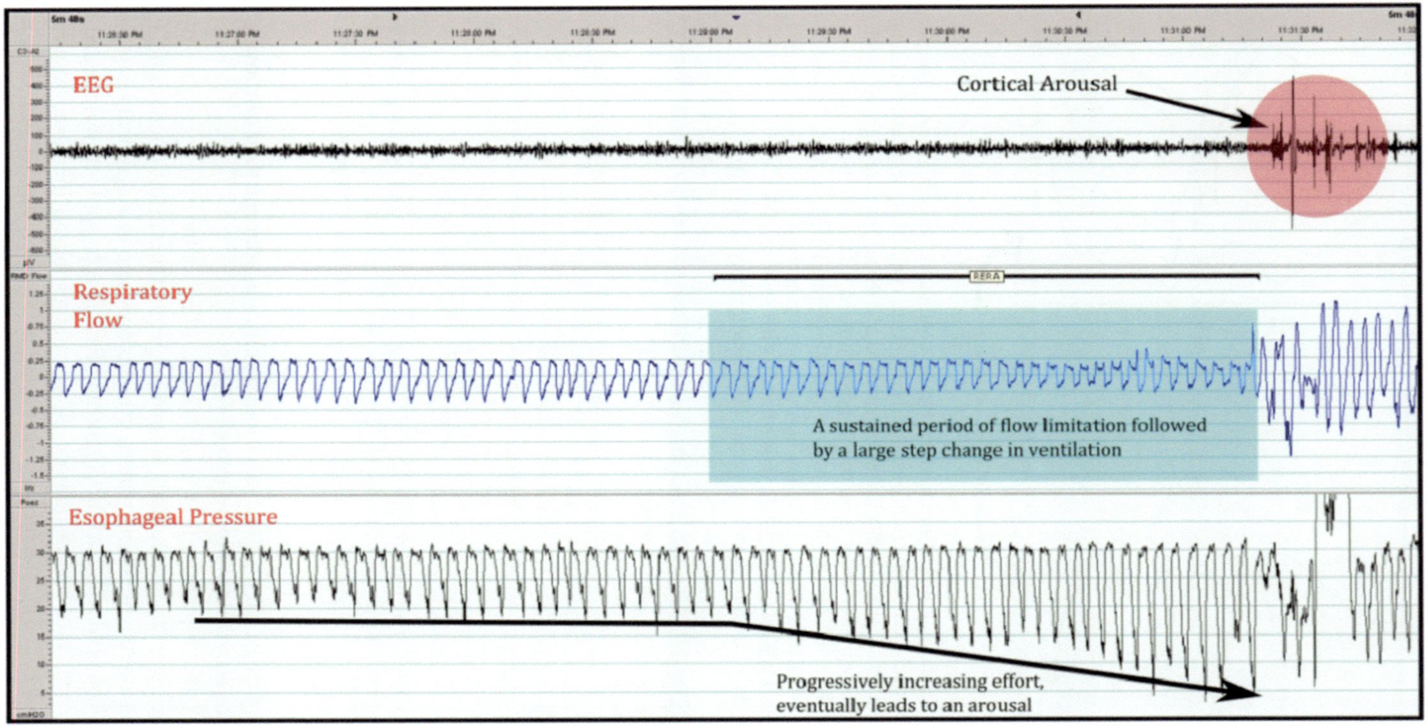

Fig. 4.13 Respiratory flow curve shows the respiratory effort-related arousals (RERAs) event. Trace shows a sustained period of flow limitation leading to increasing respiratory effort and arousal typical of RERAs. *EEG* electroencephalography. (Copyright © 2016 Alison Wimms et al., with permission [20])

practiced since it is uncomfortable. Consequently, often RERA events are perceived through indirect inference (in the laboratory, by observing a subtle change in the breathing pattern, with or without snoring, but with repetitive arousals or movements) [8].

In version 2.5 of AASM's Manual for the Scoring of Sleep and Associated Events: Rules, Terminology and Technical Specifications (2018), reporting RERA events remains optional, however, if presentation of the record is defined, the events must be accounted for through the detection of increased respiratory effort or by observing the flattening of the respiratory flow curve for a period of time greater than 10 s, resulting in arousal, but without fulfilling criteria that allow classifying this event as another respiratory sleep disorder (apnea or hypopnea) (Fig. 4.14).

The occurrence of multiple episodes of upper airway resistance without frank apneas means that an AHI value may not provide a physician with a true indication of the degree of sleep fragmentation being experienced by patients. Correcting RERA event is very important, as several studies have already shown that even a limitation in respiratory flow can lead to increased sleepiness, cardiovascular changes, and damage to health in general (Fig. 4.15) [12].

The RERA detector on PAP devices measures the number of events that interfere with patients' breathing during sleep. The scoring of an RERA requires a minimum of two limited flow breaths (flat or M-shaped) and a reduction in the magnitude of these breaths. This is important as many short apneas may not make the threshold to be identified and logged as an apnea or hypopnea, and hence are overlooked in the overall assessment of sleep quality. It also alerts clinicians to the presence of residual respiratory problems and the need to modify treatment (Fig. 4.16).

4.1.5 *Periodic Breathing*

Generally, when apnea events are observed at respiratory flow curves, it is not uncommon to see respiratory patterns that suggest periodic breathing. This phenomenon is frequently observed in central sleep apnea emerging from treatment, Cheyne-Stokes respiration (CSR), after stroke and in mixed apnea events. However, it is interesting to note that periodic respirations exhibit a different morphology when analyzing the respiratory flow curve, depending on the pathophysiology of the event (Fig. 4.17) [22].

Periodic breath algorithm detection can further improve the effective management of pressure therapy by providing additional clinical information. The periodic breathing detection algorithm measures multiple aspects of the patient's respiratory flow, including tidal volume signal for each breath, to determine apneas and hypopneas, and a sign of new inspirations and expirations beginning. Key characteristics include the length of each cycle, the amplitude of each breath, and the shape of the flow curve (of each breath) (Fig. 4.18).

Periodic breathing can be defined by the algorithm as CSR if both situations are encountered: 1. episodes of at least three consecutive central apneas and/or central

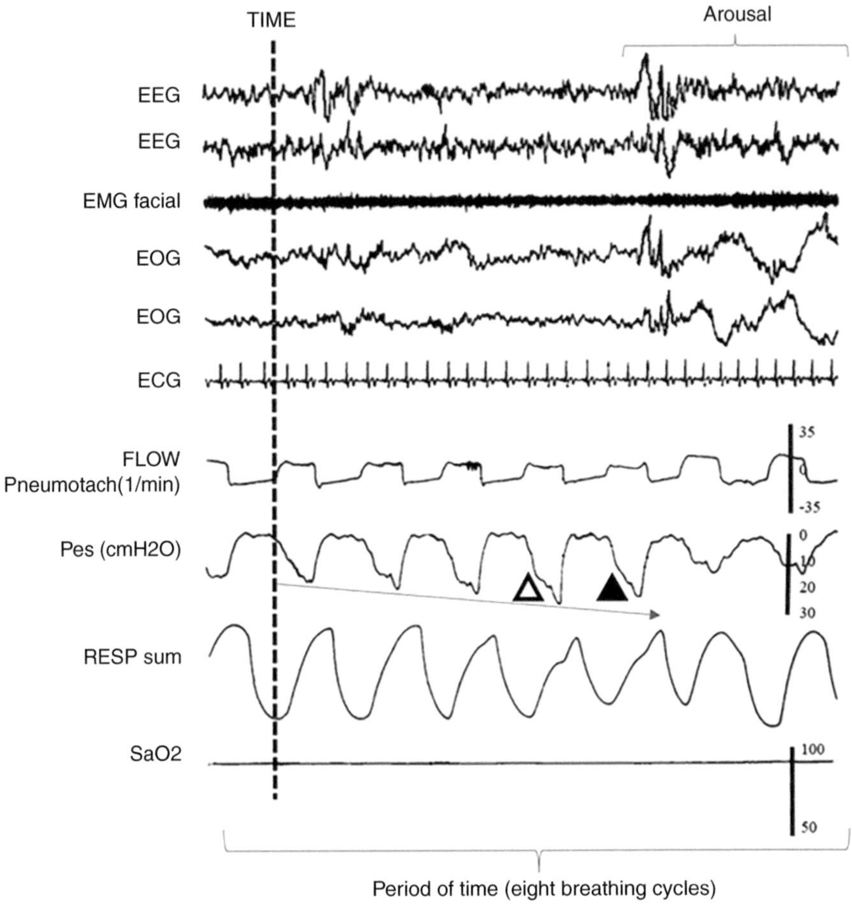

Fig. 4.14 Monitoring of an alpha electroencephalography (EEG) arousal with quantitative evaluation of airflow. Flow is measured with a tightly fitting mask and a heated pneumotachograph. Esophageal pressure (Pes) is at its nadir in the two breaths just preceding the arousal (indicated by triangles). The arousal begins with the second Pes nadir. Immediately following the onset of the transient arousal, inspiratory Pes nadir is less negative (breath just following black triangle). The "sum" signal of inductive respiratory plethysmography presents some change in shape. However, this change would be difficult to interpret if flow and Pes were not simultaneously measured. No desaturation is noted in the pulse oximetry recording. The flow decreased the most in the breath just preceding the arousal (black triangle) but is already decreasing in the breath marked by the white arrow. (Modified from Guilleminault et al., 1993 (with permission) [21])

hypopneas separated by "crescendo-decrescendo" breaths, with changes in cycle amplitude during at least 40 seconds (typically 45–90 s); 2. presence of five or more central apneas and/or central hypopneas per hour associated with a "crescendo-decrescendo" pattern recorded for at least 2 h of monitoring, for a minimum of 15 min of duration (Fig. 4.19) [23].

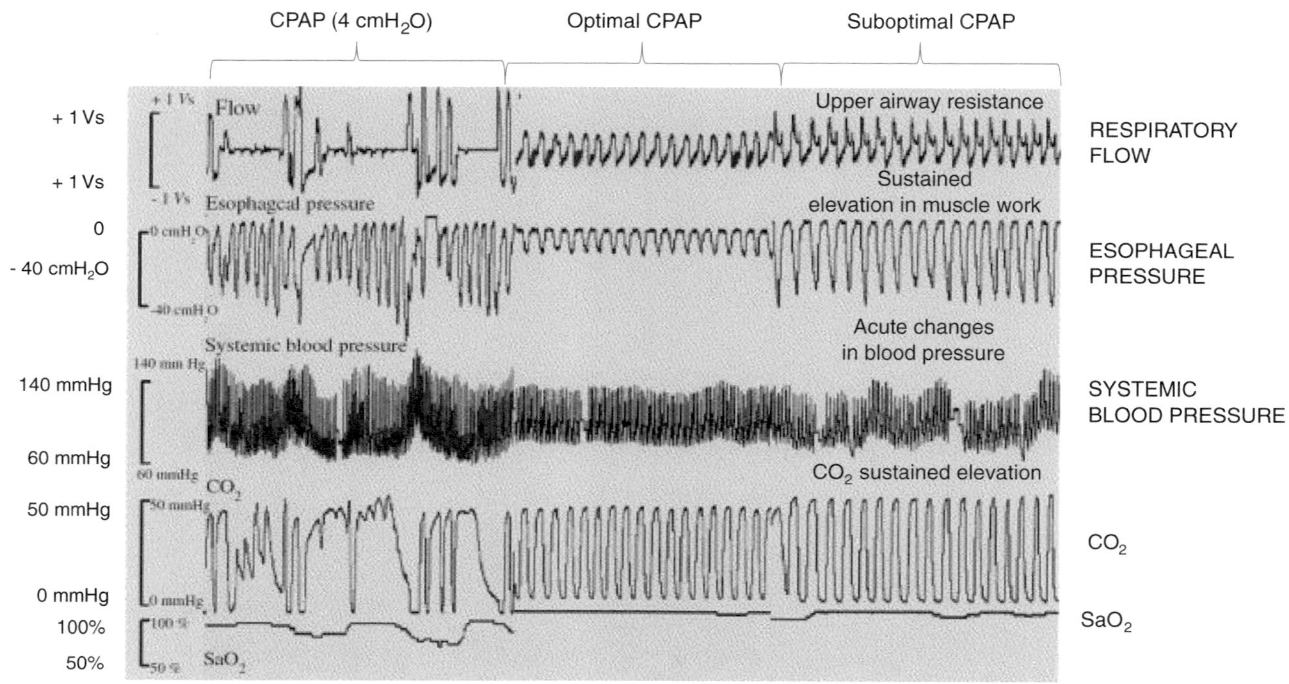

Fig. 4.15 In this figure, we see three different CPAP levels applied to the same individual. At a pressure of 4 cmH_2O (sham CPAP), apneas are present; at the optimum CPAP level the flow curve is normalized; at the sub-therapeutic level, limitations in the respiratory flow curve are observed, with an increase in EtCO2, fluctuations in blood pressure and variations in esophageal pressure (as occurs in the sham CPAP). (Source: Modified from Calero et al., 2006 (with permission) [12])

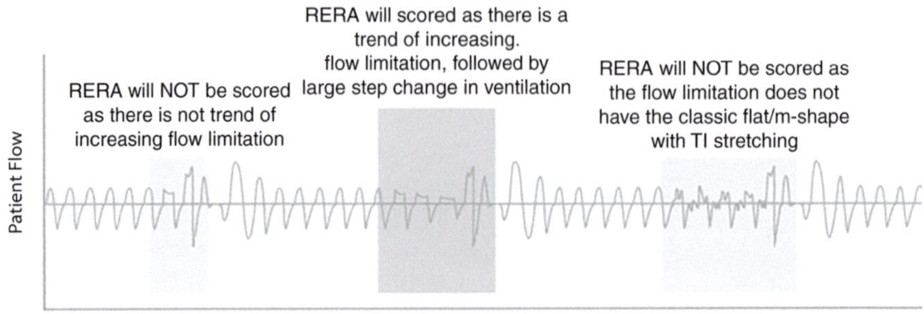

Fig. 4.16 Schematic of ResMed's algorithm for detecting respiratory effort related arousals (RERA). The scoring of an RERA requires a minimum of two limited flow breaths (flat or M-shaped) and a reduction in the magnitude of these breaths. (Figure Copyright ResMed (with permission))

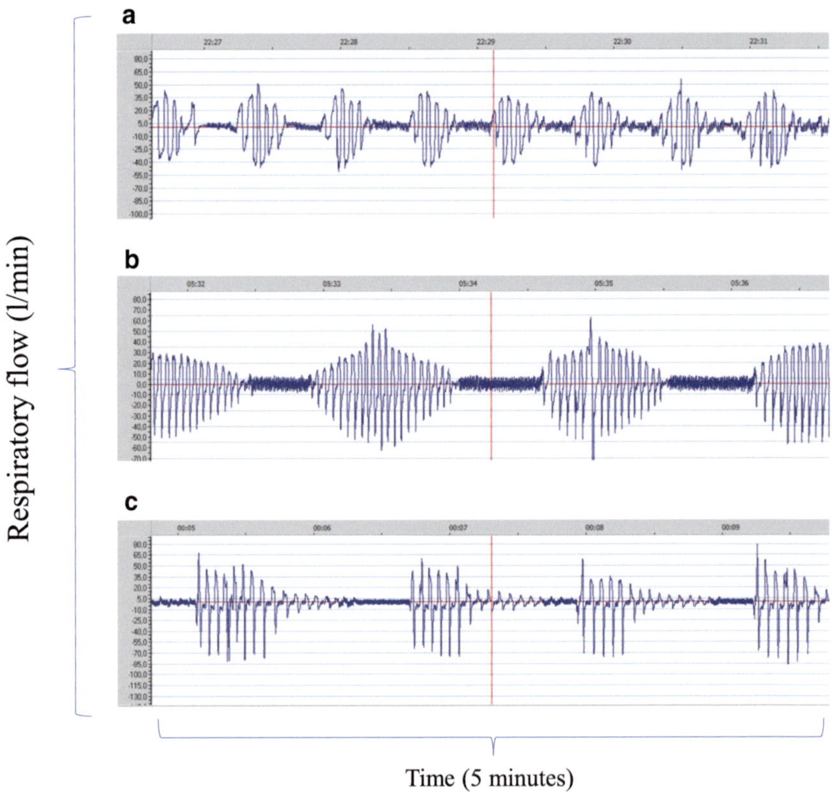

Fig. 4.17 This figure shows examples of different patterns of periodic breaths: (**a**) respiratory pattern commonly seen after stroke or in neurological diseases, with short respiratory cycles in "crescendo-decrescendo" intercut with short periods of apnea or hypopnea; (**b**) Cheyne-Stokes breathing pattern, where the respiratory cycles have a "diamond" shape, in "crescendo-decrescendo" pattern, are prolonged apneas; (**c**) more observed in mixed apneas, when the apnea event is followed by a great inspiratory movement to "open" the upper airway and to restore breathing (probably due to a microarousal). Source: author's collection

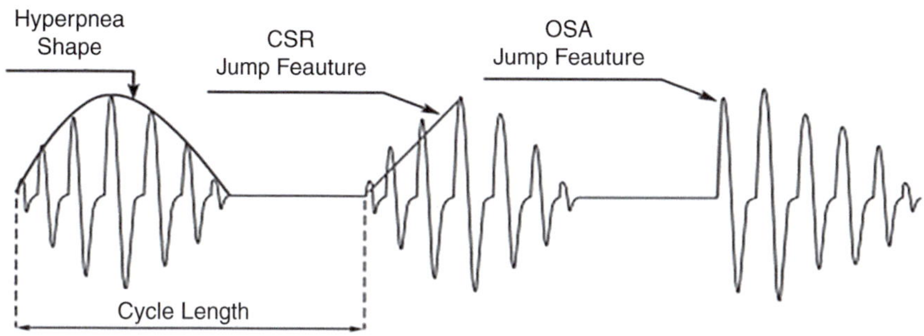

Fig. 4.18 ResMed algorithm diagram for detecting Cheyne-Stoke respiration (CSR). To detect the presence or absence of CSR, the algorithm looks for: cycle length (should be between 40 and 120 s of periodic breathing), respiratory flow curve form of the hyperpnea event and a "jump feature" (which numerically represents the ventilatory drive rate return after an apnea or hypopnea). The ventilation return differs distinctly between CSR and periods of obstructive sleep apnea, providing an excellent way to distinguish between these respiratory events. (Figure Copyright ResMed (with permission))

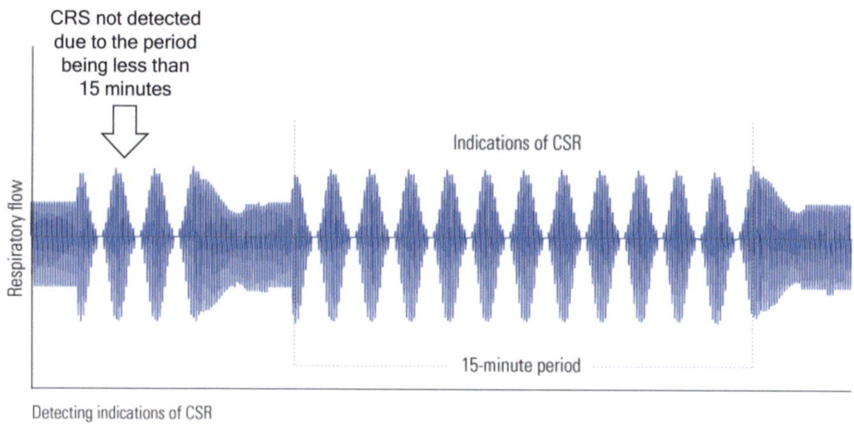

Fig. 4.19 Schematic of the ResMed algorithm to detect periodic respiration. CSR: Cheyne-Stoke respiration. (Figure Copyright ResMed (with permission))

For CSR detection, a period of 90 min of respiratory flow (consecutive epochs) is analyzed. At least 15 min of each epoch must contain "crescendo-decrescendo" respiratory cycles for the CSR to be identified (which typically occurs in blocks of 15–30 min). Each increasing-decreasing cycle is identified as "CSR" or "non-CSR" by the PAP algorithm. If more than 50% of the epoch is identified as CSR-type, the algorithm will score "CSR.

Often, normal people may have some level of periodic breathing at sleep onset, but this does not necessarily mean that they have CSR. The ResMed algorithm looks at a long period of time, thus avoiding false positive cases (a typical CSR patient has a 45–90 s cycle, and at 90 s, 10 cycles correspond to 15 min). ResMed algorithm showed a specificity of 90% over 70 studies and a negative predictive ratio of 0.2 [23].

As mentioned above, central sleep apnea emerging from treatment may also present a respiratory pattern suggestive of periodical breathing. Called treatment-emergent central sleep apneas (TECSA), distinguishing this phenomenon by analyzing the respiratory airflow curve can be challenging.

TECSA is a specific form of sleep-disordered breathing, characterized by the emergence or persistence of central apneas during treatment for obstructive sleep apnea (but it can also occur because of other OSA treatment, such as the use of a mandibular advancement device (MAD), maxillomandibular advancement surgery, sinus and nasal surgery, and tracheostomy) [24]. The respiratory flow curve differs from that observed in Cheyne-Stokes breathing and the periodic breathing pattern is not very homogeneous. Often, the central events are crossed by "attempts" to restore normal respiration, probably triggered by the respiratory center (Fig. 4.20).

4.1.6 *Snore Index (Vibrating Airway)*

Snoring is the sound generated by vibrations of the walls of the upper airway. It is generally, but not always, preceded by flow limitation or a partial obstruction of the airway.

The ResMed algorithm identifies true snores by measuring oscillations in the pressure curve. It calculates the severity of a snore based on a single breath, then (in automatic devices) responds to snoring after the first occurrence for quick and accurate resolution. For automated machines, the ResMed algorithm (AutoSet™) provides a pressure response based on the degree of oscillation or the severity of snoring (increases the pressure relative to the severity of snoring). Increases pressure in

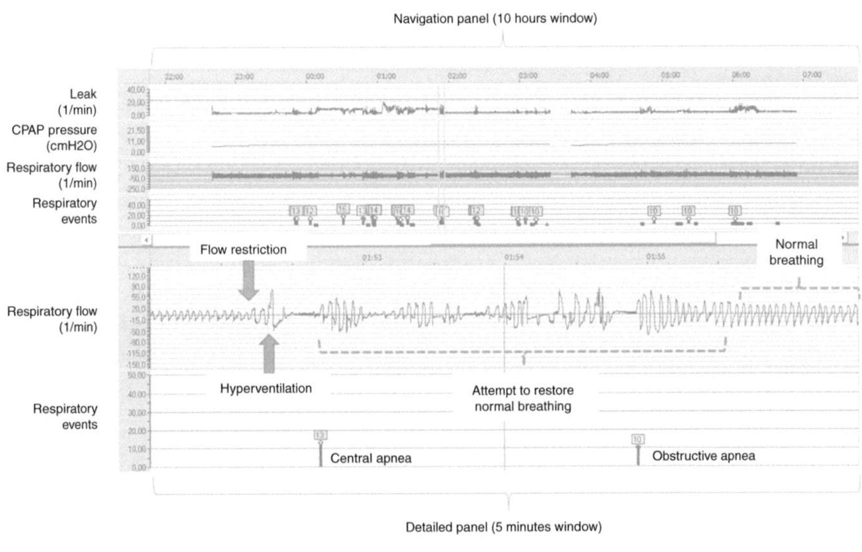

Fig. 4.20 Respiratory flow curve pattern of treatment-emergent central sleep apnea. Observe the heterogeneous flow curve change in the patient's breathing pattern as an attempt to restore normal breathing, after a central apnea event. (Source: author's collection)

relation to the loudness of the snore (up to 0.2 cmH_2O/s for snores that register above 0.2 snore units). It responds to events based on a multiple-breath moving average of the inspiratory flow-time curve in order to prevent the device from responding to random breathing events, such as sighs or coughs.

In addition, the algorithm filters out fluctuations due to deep breaths. It does this by looking at the current breath versus the average of ventilation of the previous 3 min. If the breath is too large (characteristic of a snore), the device will filter out the aberration signal and will know not to respond.

The ResMed algorithm takes the calculations for the most recent breaths, averages them, and determines whether to respond. If a response is needed, it calculates the appropriate response and increases or decreases pressure accordingly. When the patient takes the next breath, the device does the same thing—it adds in the most recent breath, drops the oldest one, creates a new average, and responds as needed.

It is important to note that ResMed machines do not use a microphone to capture an audio signal. Microphones can capture trivial environmental sounds. By reacting to changes in the pressure curve caused by snoring disturbances, the algorithm makes sure that the responses are appropriate.

In non-automatic devices the snoring index can give us valuable information to adjust the patient's pressure level. Often in the statistical report, the AHI is normalized, but when we check the Snore Index, the patient is snoring. In these cases, a small pressure adjustment can be sufficient to normalize the respiratory flow curve and eliminate snoring (Fig. 4.21).

Sometimes, in order to see the snoring signal properly at ResScan™, you need to "give a good visual space" for this graphical signal. Place the mouse cursor between the split line on the navigation window and the detail window. Click, hold, and drag the window up. You will then see the low, moderate, and loud snoring icons (as long as you have properly selected this graph option for your screen) (Fig. 4.22).

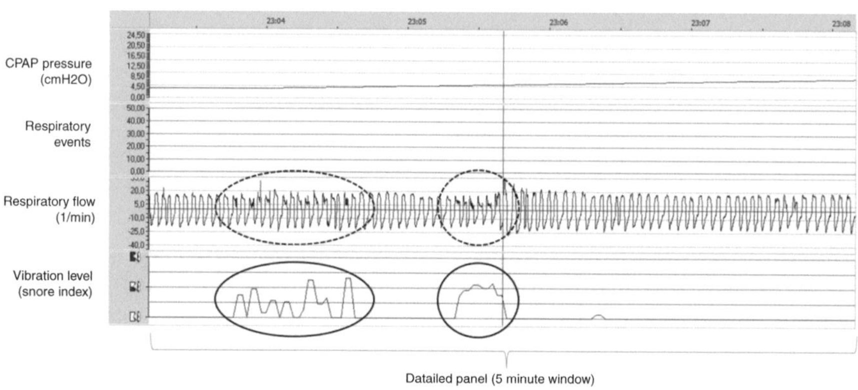

Fig. 4.21 Note in this figure that at the beginning of CPAP use, at ramp pressure, there is a respiratory flow limitation (dotted circle) and the snore icon indicates if there is a greater or lesser "snoring" (closed circle). No respiratory event is signalized at the respiratory events windows. (Source: author's collection)

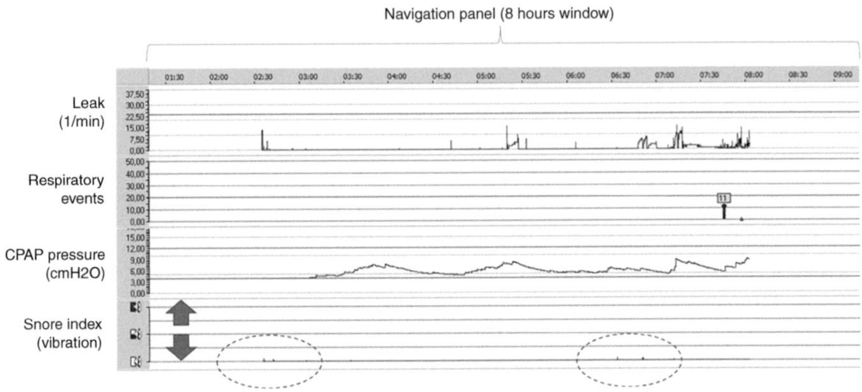

Fig. 4.22 Always visualize the snore window by opening the plot. Viewing this window with a tiny zoom can hide the presence of the snoring signal. (Source: author's collection)

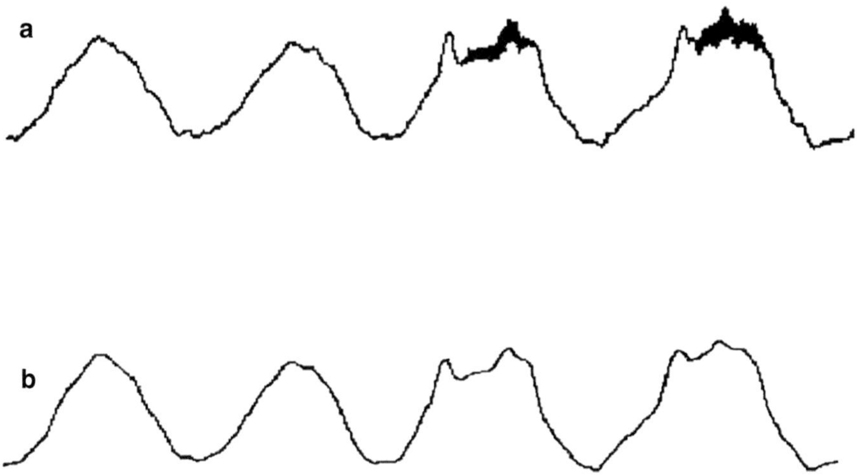

Fig. 4.23 Respiratory flow curve plotting without a filter, showing a snoring/vibration signal (**a**) and a high-frequency filter adjustment between 5 and 15 Hz, thus removing the snoring signal (**b**). (Modified after Rapoport et al., 2001 (with permission) [25])

When properly collected, the pressure curve data (unfiltered) provides more information than the simple possibility of deriving the respiratory flow curve. Breathing causes small changes in the pressure signal and, according to the filter that will be applied to the generated signals, we can show only the respiratory flow curve or even snoring events (Fig. 4.23). The reliability of the snoring signal captured by the pressure sensor in the PAP equipment cannot be compared with a microphone or a snoring sensor. However, this information is very useful in practice and has the advantage of not being contaminated by noise from the environment (but it can be contaminated by increasing the resistance to the passage of airflow in the circuit through condensation, for example).

4.2 Other Information from the Detailed Graphs

Other advanced graphic information is detailed here, which also helps us to better assess the patient using pressure therapy to treat sleep-related breathing disorders. The illustrations in this section have been adapted from ResMed technical training material and images from the ResScanTM screen in the author's collection.

4.2.1 *Unintentional Leak*

In ResMed devices, it measures unintentional leakage events in one overnight assessment. Refers to involuntary leakage (i.e., the leak value after deducting the intentional leak from the mask). The idea is that the leak should be less than 24 L/min throughout the night using nasal interfaces and less than 36 L/min using oronasal interfaces (values exclusive to ResMed's equipment). A high level of leakage can interfere with data accuracy (Fig. 4.24).

4.2.2 *Pressure*

The pressure graph provides an opportunity to examine pressure increases in response to respiratory events. When the airway is not obstructed, the pressure starts to decrease, which is graphically represented (Fig. 4.25).

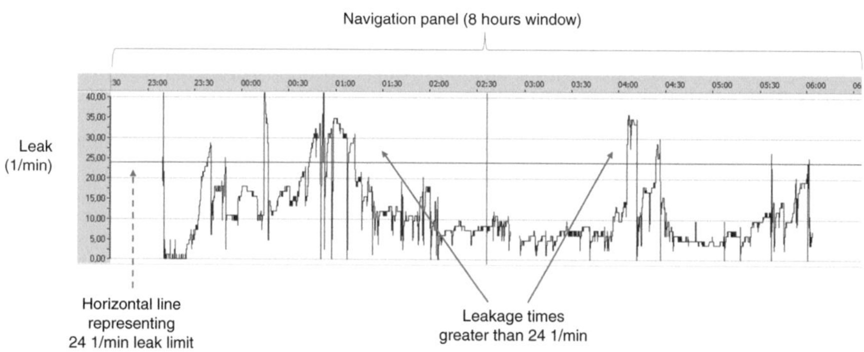

Fig. 4.24 The periods of increased leakage extrapolate the upper line of the figure which, in the ResScan™ system, determines the cut-off point of 24 L/min. Visualization of the leak curve graphics allows verification of the distribution of excessive leakage overnight. (Source: author's collection)

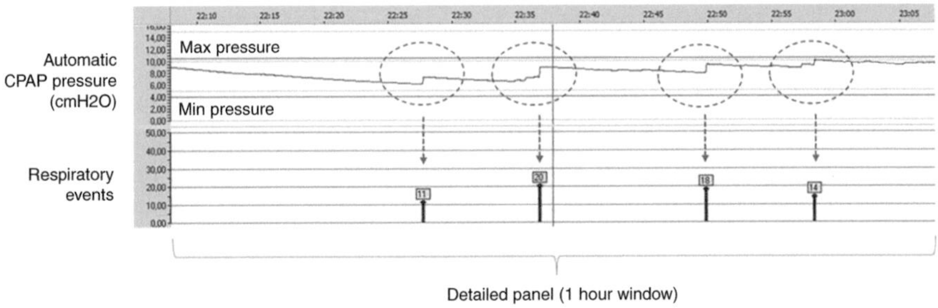

Fig. 4.25 This figure shows that in case of obstructive events, the AutoSet™ algorithm shows an increase in pressure. In the PAP automatic mode, after a period of respiratory flow stability, the therapeutic pressure decreases (the algorithm works to maintain the lowest and most effective therapeutic pressure to maintain upper airway patency during sleep). (Source: author's collection)

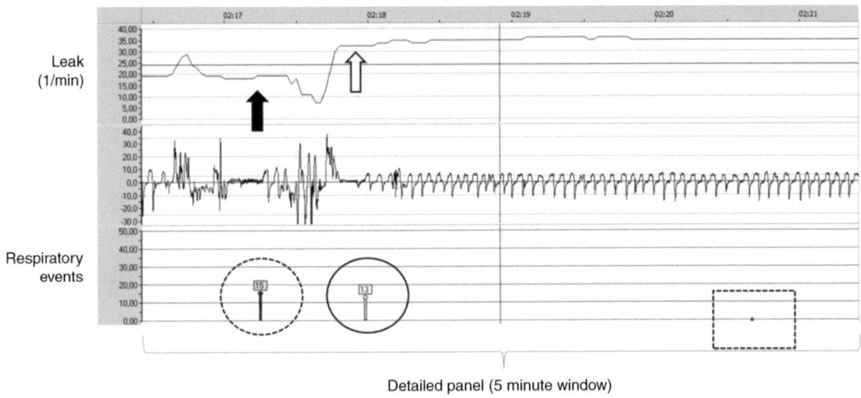

Fig. 4.26 This figure shows the tagging of breathing events. Obstructive apnea of 15 seconds duration (dotted circle); unknown apnea of 13 seconds durations (closed circle), and RERA event (dotted square). Note that the unknown apnea occurred at a greater leakage (open arrow), and the obstructive apnea event was recognized by the algorithm because the leak was not so high (closed arrow). Source: author's collection

4.2.3 Events

Refer to unusual respiratory patterns which are recorded as events. Superior PAP devices can record events such as RERA, hypopnea, central and obstructive apnea, concomitant with the respiratory flow curve. So far, devices do not distinguish between central and obstructive hypopnea, or mixed apnea.

In ResScan™ events are color-coded according to type (central apnea in purple, obstructive apnea in red, unknown apnea (which cannot be defined because it occurs in the presence of high unintentional leak: > 0.5 L/s or 30 L/min) in yellow, hypopnea in blue (square signal) and RERA in green (triangle signal). The number above the apnea event tag (central, obstructive, or unknown) indicates the duration of the apnea, in seconds (Fig. 4.26).

4.3 Oximeter Adapter Coupled to the PAP Device

Oxygen desaturation (SpO_2) obtained by night pulse oximetry is an important parameter in sleep medicine, mainly for the diagnosis of respiratory problems during sleep. In addition, the evaluation of nocturnal oximetry concomitant with the use of the pressure therapy device can help the health professional to make therapeutic adjustments in specific cases (e.g., obesity hypoventilation, COPD, etc.).

On compatible ResMed machines, the oximeter adapter connects a NONIN Xpod™ oximeter with the PAP unit (Fig. 4.27). The oximeter adapter enables the device to capture and record pulse oximetry data (SpO_2, pulse rate, oxygen desaturation index) on the SD card. The data can be viewed on a telemonitoring platform or by downloading the SD data card to the software. Oxymetry is not stored in the device. It works in therapy mode when the patient is breathing through the mask. Also, it allows to record the saturation and pulse of the patient for 30 nights.

As an additional information, if the addition of supplemental oxygen to the PAP device is necessary, at a fixed rate of supplemental oxygen flow the inhaled oxygen concentration will vary depending on the pressure settings, patient breathing pattern, mask selection, and the leak rate. To connect supplemental oxygen to the device, you need to connect an oxygen connector port. The addition of oxygen may affect the pressure provided and the accuracy of the displayed leak and minute ventilation. Before adding oxygen, be familiar with the cautionary statements about using supplemental oxygen.

4.3.1 *Wireless High-Resolution Oximeter*

The overnight pulse oximetry test is a common screening test that assesses oxygen levels in the blood. When an oximeter adapter is not available, another option for measuring night oximetry at the same time as the use of the pressure therapy device is the high-resolution wireless oximeter. The Biologix® is a wireless high-resolution oximeter device that scores all desaturations of at least 3% of the baseline,

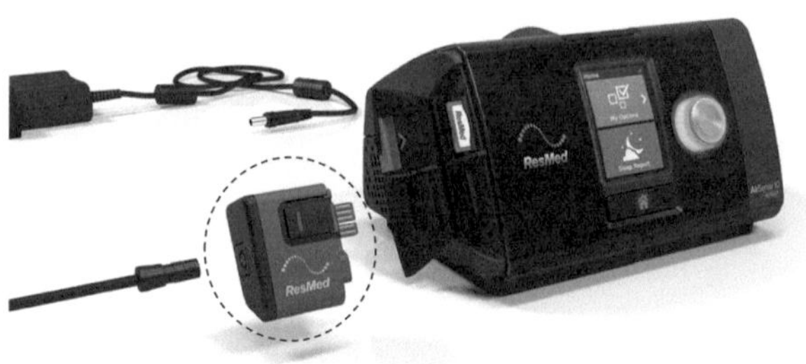

Fig. 4.27 The oximeter adapter (dotted circle) is connected to an oximetry sensor (disposable or finger sleeve model), which in turn is connected to the patient's finger during sleep, while using the positive pressure device. (Figure Copyright ResMed (with permission))

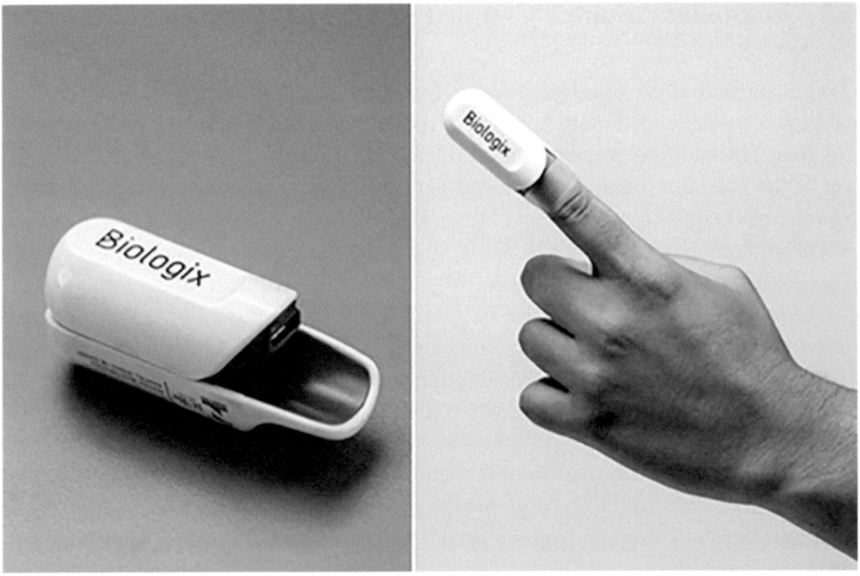

Fig. 4.28 Figure ©Biologix (with permission)

calculating both the desaturation rate and the time the patient's saturation stays below 90%. Although this equipment does not record desaturation concomitantly with the respiratory flow curve (as the oximeter adapter that was showed before), it can be of great value to indirectly assess ventilation during sleep in patients with ventilatory disorders associated with OSA. This is an option that should be considered, especially as regards its low cost (Fig. 4.28).

4.4 Further Reading

Additional information on pressure device algorithms for sleep-disordered breathing treatment can be found at McArdle N et al., 2015 (Study of a Novel APAP Algorithm for the Treatment of Obstructive Sleep Apnea in Women) [26]. Also interesting information about this new tool, the wireless high-resolution oximeter, can be found at Hasan R et al., 2022 (Validation of an overnight wireless high-resolution oximeter for the diagnosis of obstructive sleep apnea at home) [27].

References

1. Rundo JV, Downey R. Polysomnography. Handb Clin Neurol. 2019;160:381–92. https://doi.org/10.1016/B978-0-444-64032-1.00025-4.

2. Berry RB, Kushida CA, Kryger MH, Soto-Calderon H, Staley B, Kuna ST. Respiratory event detection by a positive airway pressure device. Sleep. 2012;35(3):361–7. https://doi.org/10.5665/sleep.1696.
3. Liu P, Chen Q, Yuan F, Zhang Q, Zhang X, Xue C, et al. Clinical predictors of mixed apneas in patients with obstructive sleep apnea (OSA). Nat Sci Sleep. 2022;14:373–80. https://doi.org/10.2147/NSS.S351946.
4. Yamauchi M, Tamaki S, Yoshikawa M, Ohnishi Y, Nakano H, Jacono FJ, et al. Differences in breathing patterning during wakefulness in patients with mixed apnea-dominant vs obstructive-dominant sleep apnea. Chest. 2011;140(1):54–61. https://doi.org/10.1378/chest.10-1082.
5. Lee SA, Lee GH, Chung YS, Kim WS. Clinical, polysomnographic, and CPAP titration features of obstructive sleep apnea: mixed versus purely obstructive type. J Neurol Sci. 2015;355(1–2):150–4. https://doi.org/10.1016/j.jns.2015.06.005.
6. Kairaitis K, Byth K, Parikh R, Stavrinou R, Wheatley JR, Amis TC. Tracheal traction effects on upper airway patency in rabbits: the role of tissue pressure. Sleep. 2007;30(2):179–86. https://doi.org/10.1093/sleep/30.2.179.
7. Squier SB, Patil SP, Schneider H, Kirkness JP, Smith PL, Schwartz AR. Effect of end-expiratory lung volume on upper airway collapsibility in sleeping men and women. J Appl Physiol (1985). 2010;109(4):977–85. https://doi.org/10.1152/japplphysiol.00080.2010.
8. Berry RBBR, Gamaldo CE, Harding SM, Marcus CL, Vaughn BV, Tangredi MM, for the American Academy of Sleep Medicine. The AASM manual for the scoring of sleep and associated events: rules, terminology and technical specifications. Darien, IL: https://www.aasmnet.org; 2012.
9. Berry RB, Budhiraja R, Gottlieb DJ, Gozal D, Iber C, Kapur VK, et al. Rules for scoring respiratory events in sleep: update of the 2007 AASM manual for the scoring of sleep and associated events. Deliberations of the sleep apnea definitions task force of the American Academy of sleep medicine. J Clin Sleep Med. 2012;8(5):597–619. https://doi.org/10.5664/jcsm.2172.
10. Randerath WJ, Treml M, Priegnitz C, Stieglitz S, Hagmeyer L, Morgenstern C. Evaluation of a noninvasive algorithm for differentiation of obstructive and central hypopneas. Sleep. 2013;36(3):363–8. https://doi.org/10.5665/sleep.2450.
11. Javaheri S, Rapoport DM, Schwartz AR. Distinguishing central from obstructive hypopneas on a clinical polysomnogram. J Clin Sleep Med. 2023;19(4):823–34. https://doi.org/10.5664/jcsm.10420.
12. Calero G, Farre R, Ballester E, Hernandez L, Daniel N, Montserrat Canal JM. Physiological consequences of prolonged periods of flow limitation in patients with sleep apnea hypopnea syndrome. Respir Med. 2006;100(5):813–7. https://doi.org/10.1016/j.rmed.2005.09.016.
13. Genta PR, Sands SA, Butler JP, Loring SH, Katz ES, Demko BG, et al. Airflow shape is associated with the pharyngeal structure causing OSA. Chest. 2017;152(3):537–46. https://doi.org/10.1016/j.chest.2017.06.017.
14. Azarbarzin A, Sands SA, Taranto-Montemurro L, Oliveira Marques MD, Genta PR, Edwards BA, et al. Estimation of pharyngeal collapsibility during sleep by peak inspiratory airflow. Sleep. 2017;40(1):zsw005. https://doi.org/10.1093/sleep/zsw005.
15. Azarbarzin A, Sands SA, Marques M, Genta PR, Taranto-Montemurro L, Messineo L, et al. Palatal prolapse as a signature of expiratory flow limitation and inspiratory palatal collapse in patients with obstructive sleep apnoea. Eur Respir J. 2018;51(2):1701419. https://doi.org/10.1183/13993003.01419-2017.
16. Azarbarzin A, Marques M, Sands SA, Op de Beeck S, Genta PR, Taranto-Montemurro L, et al. Predicting epiglottic collapse in patients with obstructive sleep apnoea. Eur Respir J. 2017;50(3):1700345. https://doi.org/10.1183/13993003.00345-2017.
17. Genta PR, Kaminska M, Edwards BA, Ebben MR, Krieger AC, Tamisier R, et al. The importance of mask selection on continuous positive airway pressure outcomes for obstructive sleep apnea. An official American Thoracic Society workshop report. Ann Am Thorac Soc. 2020;17(10):1177–85. https://doi.org/10.1513/AnnalsATS.202007-864ST.

18. Maggard MD, Sankari A, Cascella M. Upper airway resistance syndrome. Treasure Island, FL: StatPearls Publishing; 2022.
19. Ogna A, Tobback N, Andries D, Preisig M, Vollenweider P, Waeber G, et al. Prevalence and clinical significance of respiratory effort-related arousals in the general population. J Clin Sleep Med. 2018;14(8):1339–45. https://doi.org/10.5664/jcsm.7268.
20. Wimms A, Woehrle H, Ketheeswaran S, Ramanan D, Armitstead J. Obstructive sleep apnea in women: specific issues and interventions. Biomed Res Int. 2016;2016:1764837. https://doi.org/10.1155/2016/1764837.
21. Guilleminault C, Stoohs R, Clerk A, Cetel M, Maistros P. A cause of excessive daytime sleepiness. The upper airway resistance syndrome. Chest. 1993;104(3):781–7. https://doi.org/10.1378/chest.104.3.781.
22. Medicine AAoS. The international classification of sleep disorders, third edition (ICSD-3). 2014.
23. Ramanan D, Bateman P, Woehrle H, Richards G, Armitstead J. Validation of a Cheyne-stokes respiration (CSR) detection algorithm for a CPAP device. Eur Respir J. 2014;44(Suppl 58):P2007.
24. Zhang J, Wang L, Guo HJ, Wang Y, Cao J, Chen BY. Treatment-emergent central sleep apnea: a unique sleep-disordered breathing. Chin Med J. 2020;133(22):2721–30. https://doi.org/10.1097/CM9.0000000000001125.
25. Rapoport D, Norman R, Nielson M. Nasal. Pressure Airflow measurement—an introduction. Corpus Christi, TX: Pro-Tech. Services; 2001.
26. McArdle N, King S, Shepherd K, Baker V, Ramanan D, Ketheeswaran S, et al. Study of a novel APAP algorithm for the treatment of obstructive sleep apnea in women. Sleep. 2015;38(11):1775–81. https://doi.org/10.5665/sleep.5162.
27. Hasan R, Genta PR, Pinheiro GDL, Garcia ML, Scudeller PG, de Carvalho CRR, et al. Validation of an overnight wireless high-resolution oximeter for the diagnosis of obstructive sleep apnea at home. Sci Rep. 2022;12(1):15136. https://doi.org/10.1038/s41598-022-17698-8.

Chapter 5
Examples of Flow Curves and Other Advanced Graphics

In 1995, one study by Gugger et al. proved that the first ResMed algorithm developed could detect respiratory events at night. Respiratory signals were obtained by using a CPAP with the patient wearing a prong mask. The study was conducted to evaluate the accuracy of a new Continuous Positive Pressure Device (CPAP) with integrated diagnostic capabilities (Autoset™) to detect apneas. Twenty-seven patients underwent full overnight polysomnography and data with the Autoset™ were acquired simultaneously, with the patient wearing a prong mask (apneas were detected by special analysis of the flow signal). In that study the authors explained that as the Autoset™ derives all its data from one signal (respiratory flow curve derived from the oscillation of the nasal pressure signal, that occurs between the inspiratory and expiratory phases of respiration), careful examination of the raw data to assess the quality of the flow signal was essential. And, as a result, the study showed that there was a correlation between the apnea index (AI) assessed by the Autoset™ and by polysomnography AI-PSG ($r = 0.85$) and between the AI-Autoset and the apnea-hypopnoea index (AHI) during polysomnography ($r = 0.87$) [1].

Despite having the purpose of demonstrating that eventually it could be feasible to use the CPAP as a tool for identifying sleep-disordered breathing (as long as the CPAP algorithm is able to properly interpret breathing signals), the Gugger's study provided an extremely important data: the possibility of visualizing the graphic signal of the respiratory flow, provided by the CPAP itself, to confirm the veracity of the data presented by the algorithm of the pressure therapy device on the statistical report [1].

Currently, several studies have shown that it is possible, through the evaluation of the morphology of the respiratory flow curve during sleep, to identify situations such as pharyngeal collapsibility [2], palatal prolapse [3], epiglottis collapse [4], microarousals [5], recognition of the Cheyne-Stokes respiration pattern [6, 7], post-stroke sleep-disordered breathing recognition [8], and effects of positioning during sleep [9, 10], among others.

V. S. Piccin, *Monitoring Positive Pressure Therapy in Sleep-Related Breathing Disorders*, https://doi.org/10.1007/978-3-031-50292-7_5

In this chapter, we present several examples of respiratory flow curves and other high-resolution data derived from ResMed positive pressure devices, but which are also available from many other manufacturers.

5.1 Obstructive Apnea

Apnea refers to the absence (or reduction of at least 90%) of inspiratory airflow for a minimum of 10 s. An obstructive sleep apnea arises when complete upper airway occlusion occurs in the face of continued activity of inspiratory thoracic pump muscles [11].

Notice in Fig. 5.1 an obstructive apnea event, where there is a significant decrease in the respiratory flow signal, which lasts more than 10 s. After the respiratory flow obstruction interval, there is a significant increase in the inspiratory peak, which eventually could be the identification of a micro awakening in an attempt to recover the normal breathing pattern.

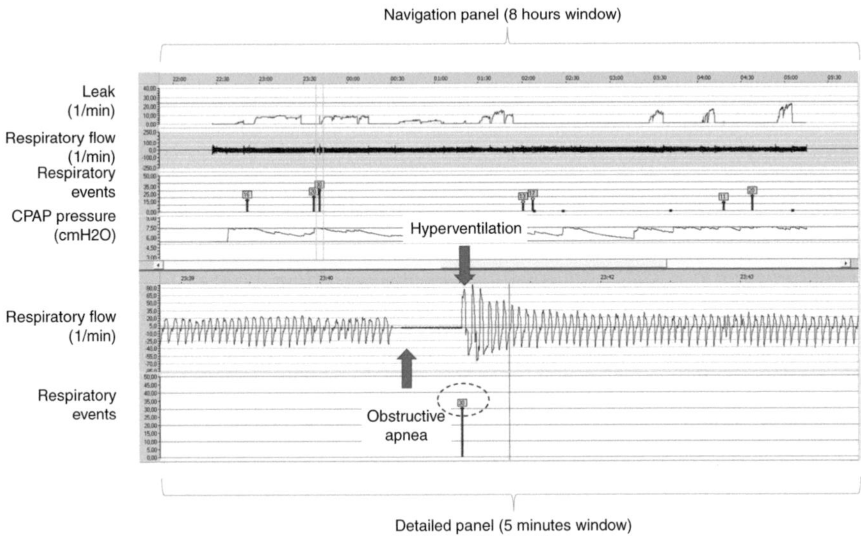

Fig. 5.1 On the detailed panel, at the respiratory flow window, there is an obstructive apnea event lasting 30 s (dashed circle) and a respiratory hyperventilation at the end of the apnea (both the obstructive apnea and hyperventilation are highlighted by closed arrows). (Source: author's collection)

5.2 Central Apnea

A central sleep apnea occurs when there is a transient reduction by the pontomedullary pacemaker in the generation of breathing rhythm, usually reflecting changes in the partial pressure of CO_2 (PCO_2), which can fall below the apneic threshold, a level of PCO_2 below which breathing ceases [11]. In the same way that obstructive apnea, in a central apnea there is also a lack (or reduction of at least 90%) of inspiratory airflow for a minimum of 10 s, but with an absence of respiratory effort during cessations of airflow.

Figure 5.2 shows the central apnea. Unlike Fig. 5.1, no significant decrease in respiratory signal can be seen before the apneic event. Instead, the event is preceded by hyperventilation, which probably caused the blood CO_2 level to drop and stimulated the central apnea response by the respiratory control center. Also note that at the end of the apnea, there is no hyperventilatory response (which often occurs in case of upper airway obstruction and subsequent microarousal).

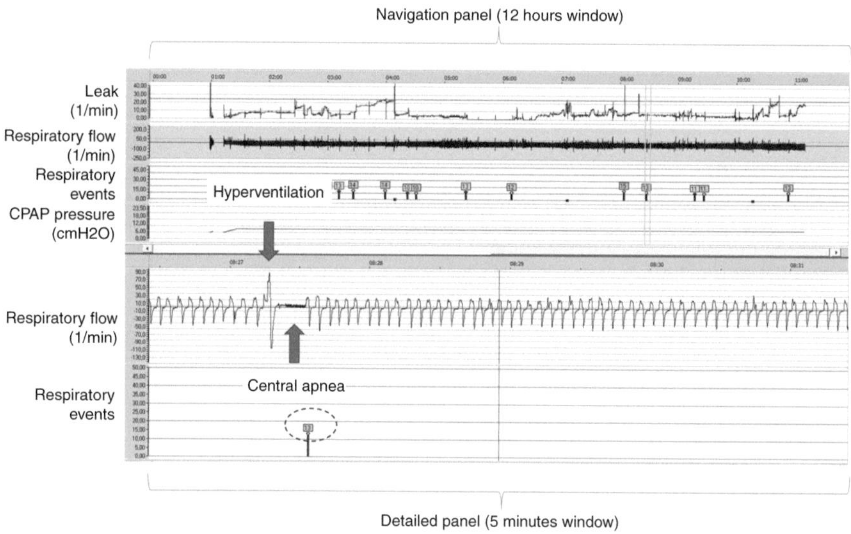

Fig. 5.2 On the detailed panel, at the respiratory flow window, there is a central apnea lasting 13 s (dashed circle). Notice the hyperventilation event at the beginning of the apnea (central apnea and hyperventilation are highlighted with closed arrows). (Source: author's collection)

5.3 Central Apnea with Cheyne-Stokes Breathing Due to Hearth Failure

Cheyne-Stokes breathing (CSR) is the most well-known breathing pattern disorder. It is a periodic irregularity of respiration, characterized by an apnea event followed by breathing that begins almost imperceptibly, increases until it becomes dyspneic, and then decreases until apnea follows the last shallow breath. It generally has an increasing and decreasing trend in tidal volume (or respiratory flow). The complete cycle between hyperpneas and apneas lasts approximately 1 min (or more) [12]. In Fig. 5.3, extracted from the ResScan high-resolution data evaluation system, the characteristic pattern of CSR can be seen.

Interestingly, when we observe the statistical report of this same case (first shown in Fig. 5.3), the residual apnea index is normal (Fig. 5.4). Indeed, CSR events were diluted overnight throughout the assessment period. Without the analysis of the respiratory flow curve, it would be difficult to identify the abnormal respiratory pattern. And, in this way, we miss the opportunity, for example, to verify that the

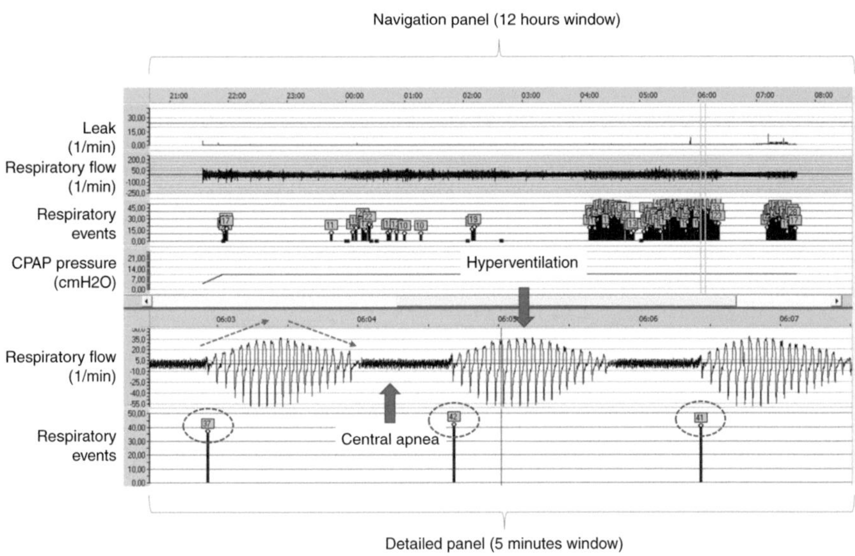

Fig. 5.3 In the respiratory flow window, in the detailed panel, some periodic breathing patterns can be observed. This periodic pattern is known as Cheyne-Stokes respiration (CSR). In CRS there is a greater amplitude and longer duration of the "crescendo-decrescendo" breathing pattern (dashed arrows), and the events of central apneas last longer, here between 37 and 42 s (dashed circle). The "crescendo-decrescendo" hyperventilation and central apnea are highlighted by closed arrows. (Source: author's collection)

Statistics

Date (report period)	Device: (model)	(S/N: --------------------)
Device Settings		
Therapy Mode: **CPAP**	EPR: **FULL TIME**	EPR Level: **3.0 cmH2O**
EPR Enable: **OFF**	EPR Patient Enable: **OFF**	Ramp Enable: **ON**
Ramp Time: **20.0 Minutes**	ESSentials: **ON**	Response: **STANDARD**
Pressure: **10.0 cmH2O**		
Leak - L/min		
Median: **0.0**	95th Percentile: **1.2**	Maximum: **7.2**
Respiratory Indices - events/hr		
Apnea Index: **2.9**	Hypopnea Index: **0.4**	AHI: **3.4**
Obstructive: **0.8**	Central: **1.7**	Unknown: **0.0**
RERA Index: **0.0**	% Time in CSR: **0.0**	
Total Usage		
Used Days >= 4 hrs : **29**	Used Days < 4 hrs : **1**	% Used Days >= 4 hrs : **96**
Days not used: **0**	Total days: **30**	Total hours used: **231: 54**
Median daily usage: **8:32**	Average daily usage: **7:43**	

Fig. 5.4 Note that in Fig. 5.3 the abnormal breathing events are concentrated in the second half of the night. When we look at the statistical report of the very same patient, the residual apnea index is 3.0 (dashed circle), which is considered normal [14]. In fact, the events are diluted throughout the period of evaluation, and the statistical report does not reliably show the patient's irregular breathing pattern. (Source: author's collection)

patient's medication is optimized or not (such as diuretics), or to take procedures to reduce the impact of liquid displacement in the rostral direction throughout the night [13] (possibly raising the head of the bed or suggesting the patient to wear compression stockings during the day), among others.

5.4 Central Apnea with Non-Cheyne-Stokes Periodic Pattern

At times, when assessing the respiratory flow curve, periodic respiratory events that do not meet the criteria of a Cheyne-Stokes respiration could be observed (Fig. 5.5). In these cases, the patient clinical history helps us to determine the event pathophysiology, which may be related, for example, to exposure to altitude [15], neurological alterations [16, 17], or even positioning during sleep [18].

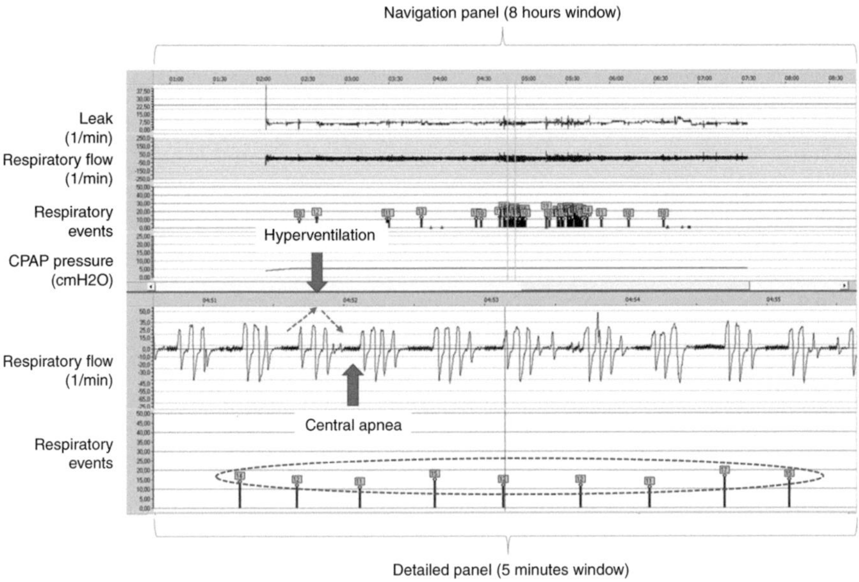

Fig. 5.5 On the detailed panel, at the respiratory flow window, a periodic breathing pattern could be observed. Unlike the Cheyne-Stokes breathing pattern, here we observed a smaller amplitude and duration of the increasing-decreasing breathing pattern (dashed arrows), and central apneas were time shorter, here lasting between 11 and 17 s (dashed circle). Both the hyperventilation in a "crescendo-decrescendo" pattern and the central apnea event are highlighted by closed arrows. (Source: author's collection)

5.5 Mixed Apneas

Mixed apneas are characterized by the absence of breathing effort and airflow in the first section (central component) of the respiratory event and breathing effort without airflow in the last section (obstructive component). Pathophysiology is based on coexisting ventilatory control instability and upper airway collapsibility [19]. Checking mixed apnea events in the airway flow curve is a challenge. Knowing the patient's medical history can be a great help in interpreting the flow curve data. But, more than that, physiology and pathophysiology knowledge about respiratory conditions and how other comorbidities may also affect the respiratory pattern is essential.

It is known that until now, the PAP algorithm does not recognize mixed apnea. If there is an apneic event, after 4 s, the algorithm will release a forced oscillation signal. If this signal returns, the event will be considered an obstructive event. In the absence of a return, the respiratory event will be identified as central.

However, in a situation where the event was of central origin, but the upper airway has collapsed due to the absence of the respiratory flow that supported it, the algorithm may inadvertently classify that event as an obstructive respiratory incident. And in this case, increased pressure by the clinician may, in turn, stimulate the onset of more central respiratory events.

Note in Fig. 5.6 that the same respiratory case is sometimes categorized as a central apnea and sometimes as an obstructive apnea.

A few hints may give us indications that a respiratory event is mixed, in the assessment of the respiratory flow curve.

For example, the same respiratory pattern is sometimes categorized as central and sometimes obstructive, as in Fig. 5.6. It is probable that events classified as obstructive are, in fact, mixed apneas.

Another example is a decreasing tendency of the airway flow curve before apnea, without flattening the airway flow curve. If the event was identified as obstructive by the algorithm, this is probably a mixed event.

A third hint is sudden hyperventilation prior to apnea. Likewise, if the event was identified as obstructive by the algorithm, it is most likely also a mixed apnea (since physiologically it is very difficult to explain the occurrence of an immediate obstructive apnea after an abrupt hyperventilation event).

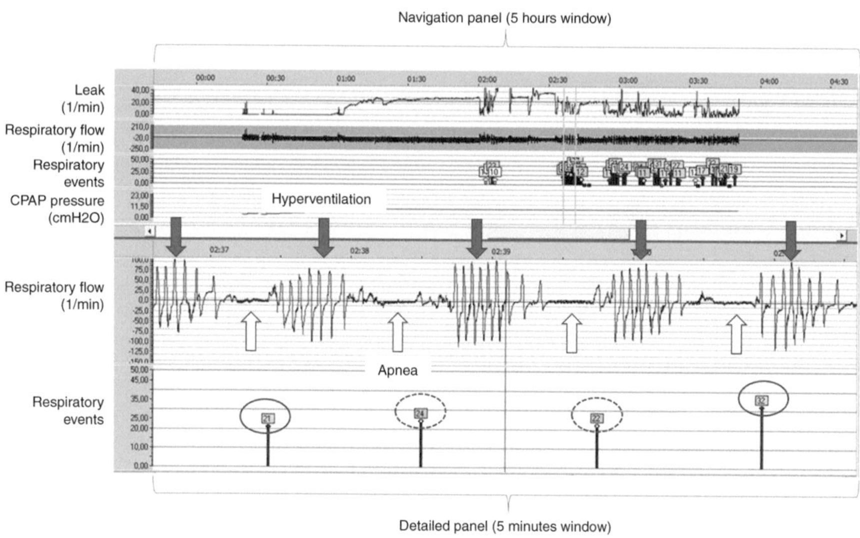

Fig. 5.6 In this figure there is a pattern of periodic breathing. At times, the algorithm classifies the same respiratory events as central apnea (dashed circle) and at times as obstructive apnea (closed circle). We highlighted the hyperventilation "crescendo-decrescendo" pattern (closed arrows) and apnea events (open arrows). (Source: author's collection)

5.6 Treatment-Emergent Central Sleep Apnea

Treatment-emergent central sleep apnea (TECSA) describes the onset of central sleep apnea (CSA) and/or central hypopnea during treatment for OSA (either by use of CPAP or mandibular advancement device, maxillomandibular advancement surgery, nose surgery and even tracheostomy). In some cases of TECSA, the occurrence of CSA events during the initial continuous titration of positive airway pressure (CPAP) is transient and may be resolved spontaneously by chronic CPAP treatment. However, some central apneas persist even with regular CPAP therapy [20].

Central apnea usually happens right away when the patient falls asleep. As a general rule, these respiratory events do not follow a specific periodical sequence. During analysis of the respiratory flow curves, we may observe an attempt by the respiratory center to establish a regular respiratory pattern (Fig. 5.7).

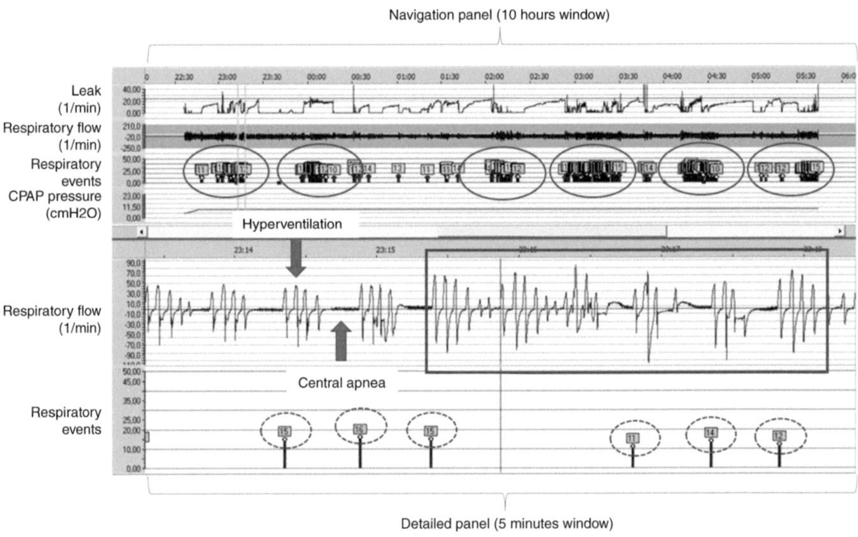

Fig. 5.7 In the detailed panel, at the respiratory flow window, some sort of periodic breathing pattern may be observed. However, it is not exactly a periodic pattern, and we can notice the change in this pattern, in an attempt by the respiratory control center to restore a more regular respiratory flow (highlighted by the open rectangle). We also observed a lower amplitude and duration of the increasing-decreasing breathing pattern and apneas (highlighted by the closed arrows). In addition, central apneas have a shorter duration; in this example they last between 11 and 16 s (dashed circle). The closed circles at the top of the navigation window highlight the periods during the night when the central apnea pattern emerging from the treatment became apparent. Note that already early in the night this configuration could be observed in the respiratory flow curve. (Source: author's collection)

5.7 Obstructive and Central Hypopnea

The American Academy of Sleep Medicine (AASM) defines apnea as a reduction in peak thermal sensor excursion by 90% of the baseline for a minimum of 10 s. Apnea is called obstructive if the inspirational effort continues or increases with time. Conversely, a central apnea is defined by no inspiratory effort. On the other hand, hypopnea is defined by the AASM as a decrease in nasal pressure signal excursion of ≥30% and an oxygen desaturation of ≥4% or a pressure decrease of ≥50% associated with an oxygen desaturation of ≥3% or an awakening [21].

While apnea can be clearly differentiated in most cases, it is often difficult to distinguish an obstructive hypopnea from a central hypopnea. Flattening of the inspiratory airflow curve, paradoxical breathing, waking position, sleep stages, and breathing pattern at the end of hypopnea may provide clues to classify hypopnea on polysomnography [22]. When using a PAP device, there is no encephalogram, respiratory effort strips, or position sensor. But it is possible to visualize the respiratory flow curve to see if there is a flattening of the respiratory flow curve or not, in addition to the decrease in its amplitude (Figs. 5.8 and 5.9).

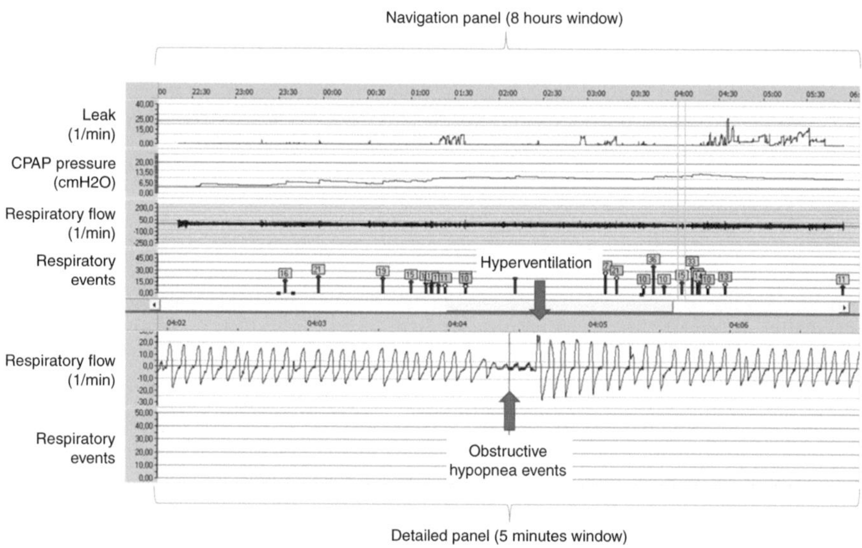

Fig. 5.8 In obstructive hypopneas, it is possible to visualize the flattening of the inspiratory flow curve. Usually, a hyperventilation event after obstructive hypopnea confirms that there has been a partial upper airway obstruction, probably followed by a microarousal. We highlight obstructive hyperventilation and hypopnea by the closed arrows, in the respiratory flow window of the detailed panel. (Source: author's collection)

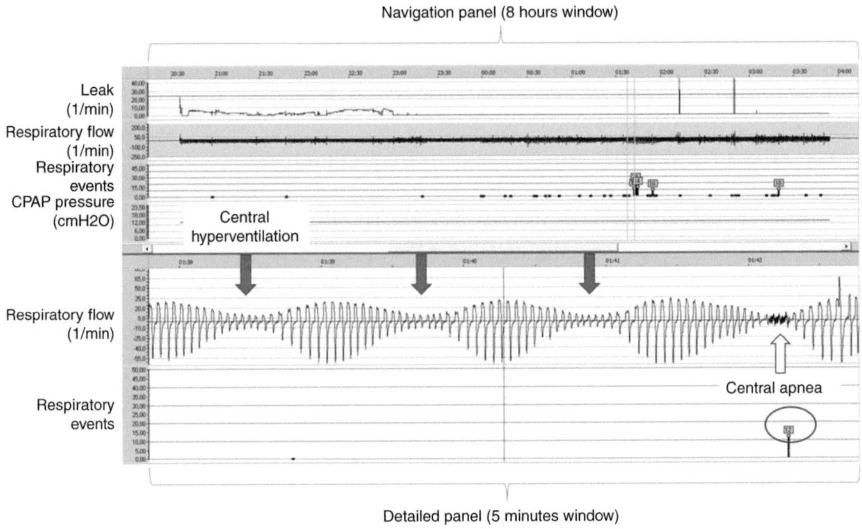

Fig. 5.9 In central hypopnea, however, there is no flattening of the inspiratory flow curve (since the decrease in respiratory flow occurred by central command and not by upper airway obstruction). Note that the respiratory flow decreases in amplitude but maintains the rounded form of the inspiratory curve (i.e., without flattening). This is a strong indication that this respiratory event is of central origin. The central hypopnea is emphasized by the closed arrows in the respiratory flow window of the detailed panel. Another interesting point to note is that the CPAP algorithm indicates only one central respiratory event in the detailed window (closed circle). (Source: author's collection)

5.8 RERA

Obstructive sleep apnea (OSA) represents the most severe form of the sleep breathing disturbances spectrum, which can be seen as a continuum, with simple snoring as its lightest form and respiratory effort related arousals (RERAs) as an intermediate feature. RERAs are characterized by respiratory events without concomitant oxygen desaturation, which may lead to daytime sleepiness and functional impairment [23]. According to the AASM Scoring Manual [24], a respiratory event can be scored as a respiratory effort-related arousal (RERA) if there is a sequence of breaths lasting ≥10 s characterized by increasing respiratory effort or by flattening of the inspiratory portion of the nasal pressure (diagnostic study) or PAP device flow (titration study) waveform leading to arousal from sleep when the sequence of breaths does not meet criteria for an apnea or hypopnea.

There are no sensors in positive pressure devices that can reliably detect an arousal. However, studies have already pointed out the expression of the respiratory flow curve that would indicate a possible awakening [5, 25]. Thus, if the equipment's algorithm detects an event that is not classified as hypopnea (but where there is an inspiratory flow curve limitation), followed by an indication of awakening (increase in the amplitude of the respiratory flow), this event will be classified as RERA (Fig. 5.10).

However, the device's algorithm can be flawed to determine events that differ slightly from one another. Note in Fig. 5.11 that for the same pattern of breathing disturbance, the algorithm sometimes differentiates between hypopneas and sometimes between RERAs. The evaluation of the flow curve is necessary for a better understanding of the residual events that the patient presents when using positive airway pressure therapy, and to conduct a more assertive therapeutic adequacy.

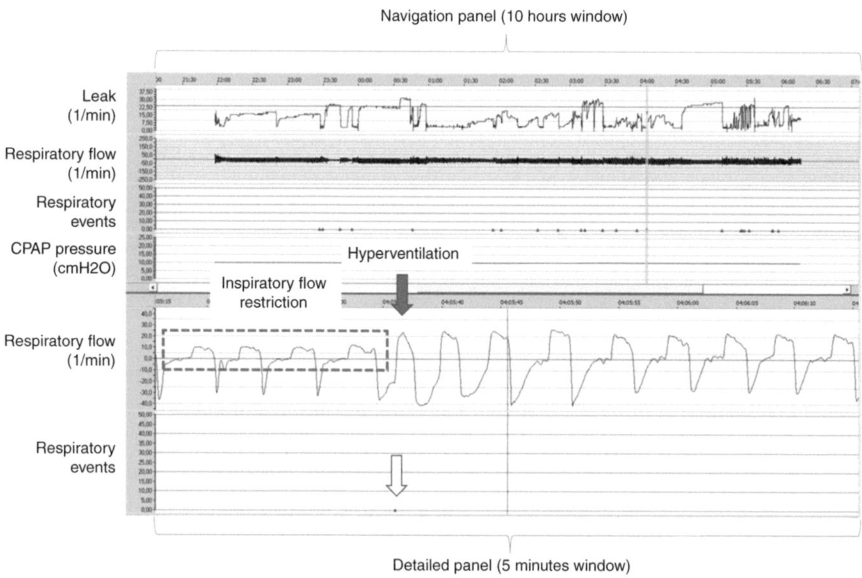

Fig. 5.10 The figure shows sequences of inspiratory flow curve limitation (dashed rectangle), followed by a significant increase in the respiratory flow curve (closed arrow), which may be an indirect indication of microarousal. The algorithm does not recognize these events as hypopneas and classifies the breathing disorder as RERA indicated by a small triangle (open arrow). (Source: author's collection)

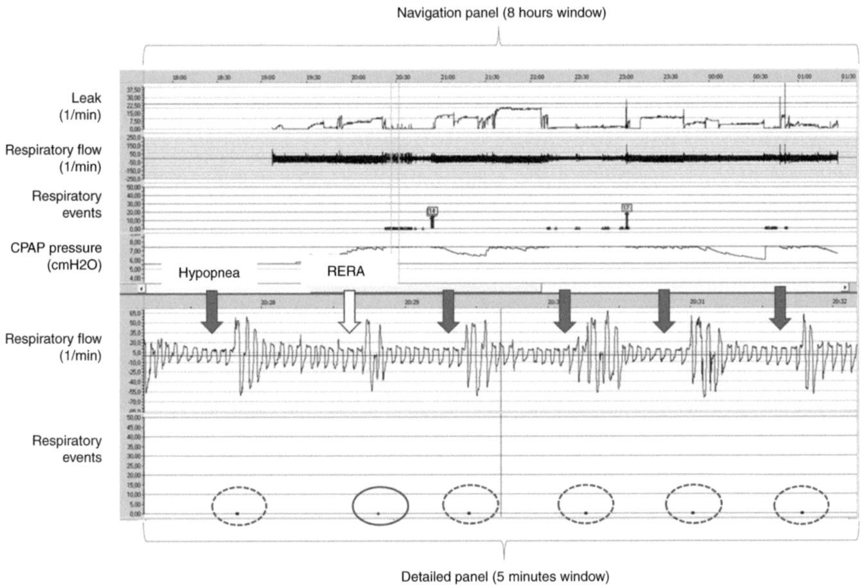

Fig. 5.11 For the same pattern of breathing disturbance (limitation of the inspiratory flow curve followed by a hyperventilation event), the algorithm makes distinctions sometimes as a hypopnea event (dashed circles and closed arrows) and sometimes as RERA event (closed circle and open arrow). (Source: author's collection)

5.9 Snore Index (Vibration Level)

The snoring index is derived from the flow-time curve and is presented as "snoring units" (vibration units or vibration level). Thus, the snoring index is a measurement based on the vibration magnitude generated by the patient's snoring.

However, the evaluation of snoring by the equipment sensor may be affected by factors such as the condensation of water in the device circuit. For example, in Fig. 5.12, we can observe the airway flow curve of a patient using a positive airway device, who has never shown any restriction in the airway flow curve or snoring. One night, there was condensation in the system circuit. That night, the increased vibration level was due to the resistance of the airflow through the water seal, not to the restriction of the airflow due to the obstruction of the upper respiratory tract.

In the example in Fig. 5.13, the patient had residual drowsiness, but the report did not show an abnormal AHI. In this specific case, despite the resolution of apnea and hypopnea events, the patient still had a flow restriction that caused snoring. The pressure increase resolved this issue, which can only be detected by evaluating the respiratory flow curve.

Figures 5.12 and 5.13 show that simply examining the vibration level signal is not enough. We must know how to interpret these data based on the patient's report, on statistical data and evaluate possible external interference.

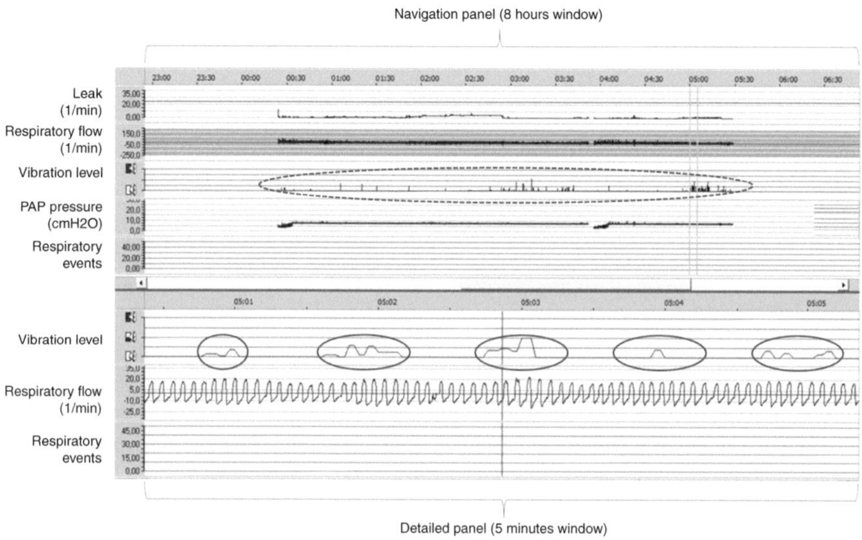

Fig. 5.12 In this figure we observe events of progressive increase in the vibration level throughout the night (dashed circle) and which are also highlighted in the detailed window (closed circles). In this occurrence, the signal was caused by the condensation of water in the positive airway pressure device circuit. (Source: author's collection)

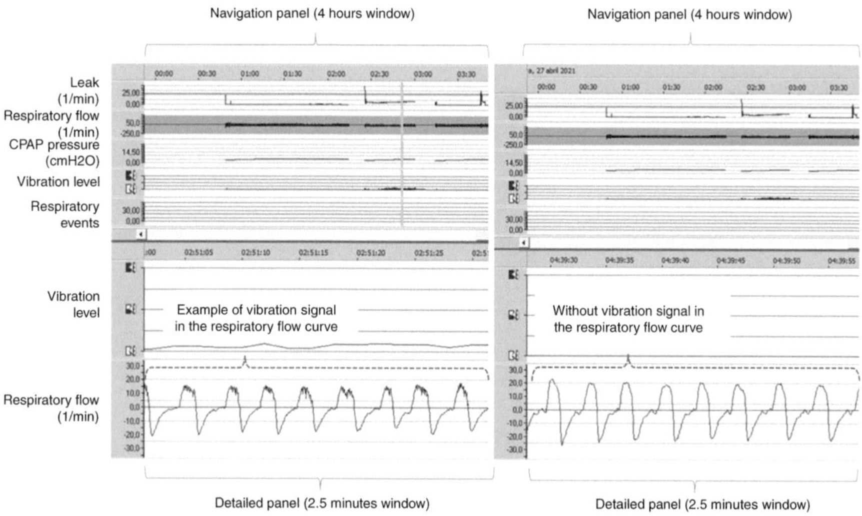

Fig. 5.13 In this example, we have two panels from the same night. In the first panel, we highlight the snoring signal in the respiratory flow curve (that increased the vibration level), where we can clearly observe the serration signal of the inspiratory flow curve presented in the detailed window. In the second panel, there is no snoring in the respiratory flow curve, and we can clearly see the correct amplitude of the inspiratory flow curve (without flow restriction). (Source: author's collection)

5.10 Breathing Pattern According to the Sleep Phase

To date, positive airway pressure devices lack sensors to identify sleep phases. However, with the knowledge of respiratory physiology, we know that the breathing pattern, when the patient is treated, is more homogeneous in the phases of NREM sleep, and more heterogeneous in REM sleep (mainly due to the emotional content of dreams) [26]. We also know that it is in REM sleep where we can find a greater decrease in muscle tone [27], which would justify the increase in therapeutic pressure in this sleep phase, when we observe the tracing of the pressure curve of a device in automatic pressure mode.

Figures 5.14 and 5.15 refer to the same patient, who has sleep apnea, who uses CPAP, with excellent therapeutic outcomes and excellent adherence to PAP. Note how indirectly we can infer, through the analysis of high-resolution graphical data, a proper recovery of the patient's sleep architecture with the use of positive airway pressure therapy.

In Fig. 5.14 we highlight in gray the periods in which there is an increase in the device pressure (navigation panel). At the same time, observe the respiratory flow curve in the detailed panel, which presents a heterogeneous trace. We may indirectly infer that the patient is in REM sleep during those times highlighted in gray.

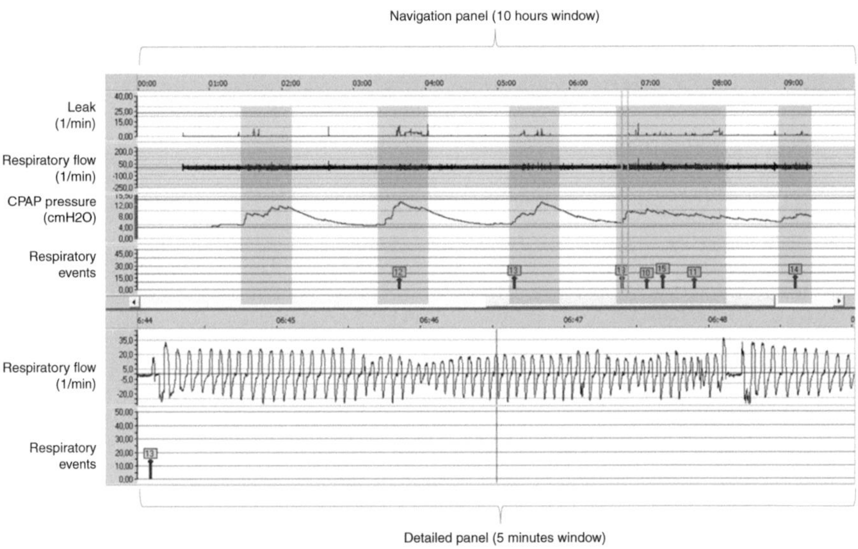

Fig. 5.14 The periods in which an increase in device pressure (navigation panel) can be observed are shown in gray. At the same time, observe the respiratory flow curve in the detailed panel, which is presenting a heterogeneous tracing, suggestive of REM stage. (Source: author's collection)

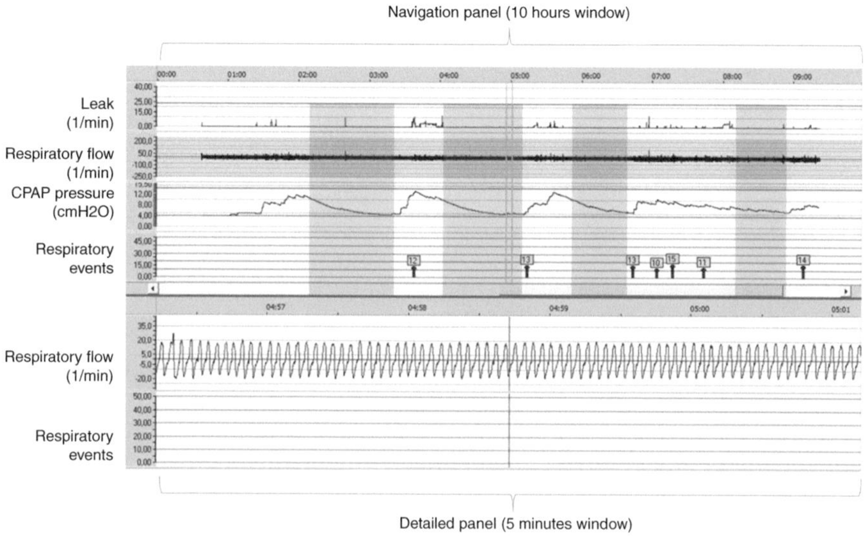

Fig. 5.15 In gray we highlight the periods in which there is a decrease in the device pressure (navigation panel). At the same time, the respiratory flow curve in the detailed panel presents a homogeneous tracing, Suggestive of NREM stage. (Source: author's collection)

In Fig. 5.15 we now highlight in gray the periods in which there is a decrease in the device pressure (navigation panel). At the same time, observe the respiratory flow curve in the detailed panel, which shows a homogenous pattern. We can indirectly infer that the patient is in NREM sleep during these periods highlighted in gray [28].

Also note that the sum of the periods of drop and rise in therapeutic pressure makes five complete "cycles". This also supports what we consider appropriate for normal sleep, which is the occurrence of 4–6 sleep cycles per night of sleep.

5.11 Loop Gain

Loop gain is a concept used to measure the stability of the chemoreflex feedback control system. The overall loop gain within the ventilatory system reflects the relationship between the ventilatory response and the disruption that caused the response (LG = ventilatory response/ventilatory disruption). Consequently, when breathing deviates from eupnea (the point where ventilation matches metabolic demand), such as during a hypopnea, if the ventilatory response that is produced is equal to the disturbance (LG = 1), ventilation will correct blood gases to re-establish eupneic

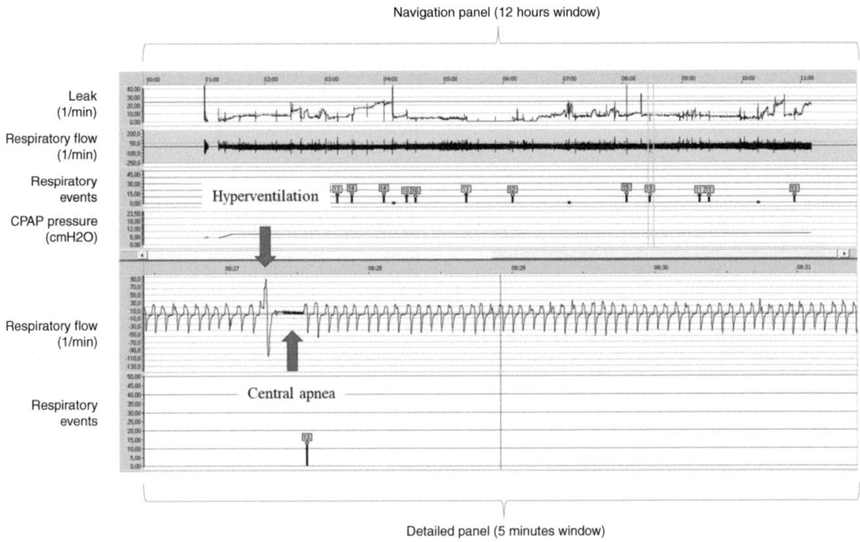

Fig. 5.16 In the analysis of the respiratory flow curve, we were able to obtain indications of the patient's phenotypic characteristic (high or low loop gain). In this figure, we can see that the patient was able to stabilize his breathing pattern after a sigh (a physiological event that leads to hyperventilation event), demonstrating the patient's phenotypic characteristic of low Loop Gain. The hyperventilation and subsequent central apnea events are highlighted by gray arrows. (Source: author's collection)

levels (Fig. 5.16). If the ventilatory response is excessively larger than the disturbance (LG > 1), ventilation will not only correct the disturbance to blood gases but will overshoot such that $PaCO_2$ will be reduced below eupneic levels (Fig. 5.17). The resulting hypocapnia will then induce hypoventilation, upper airway muscle hypotonia, and a secondary airway obstruction (apnea or hypopnea depending on succeeding upper airway mechanics), such that respiratory events become self-prolonging. Thus higher loop gain reflects less stable ventilatory chemoreflex control [29].

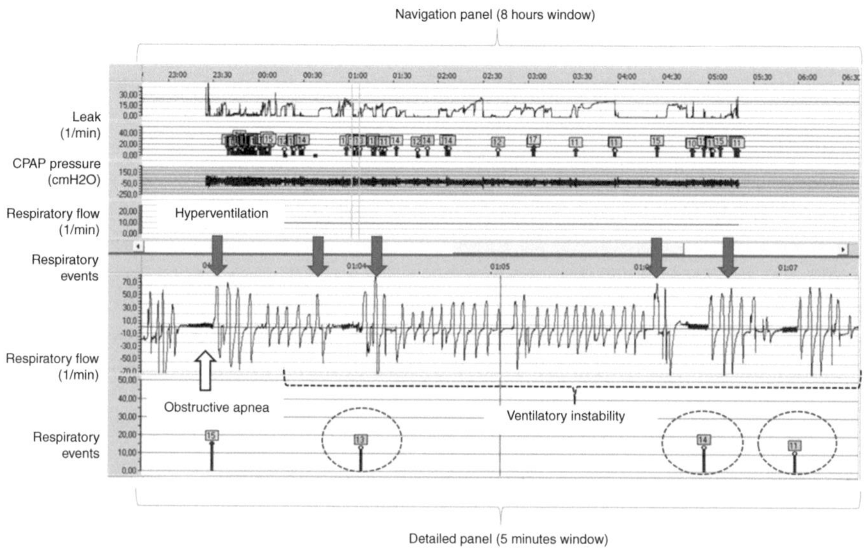

Fig. 5.17 Patients with high Loop Gain may develop cyclic events of hyperventilation and hypoventilation, stimulated by an initial stimulus (which may be, for example, a sigh or even an event of apnea, hypopnea, or increased resistance of the upper airway), maintaining these abnormal cycles for extended periods. In this figure, the patient has difficulty returning to a normal breathing pattern after an initial obstructive apnea, indicating the patient's phenotypic characteristic of high loop gain. The hyperventilation events are highlighted by gray arrows. Obstructive apnea is highlighted by the open arrow and the following central apneas are highlighted by dashed circles. (Source: author's collection)

5.12 Unintentional Leak

At ResMed sleep PAP devices, leakage refers to an unintentional leakage, which is the leakage value after deducting the intentional leakage from the mask. Maximum leak is the highest value reached during treatment. The 95th percentile leakage value is the value exceeded during the selected range for 5% of CPAP usage. This value excludes very high leakage values that are not necessarily representative of the actual clinical experience. The median leak value, recorded within the selected range, minimizes the impact of extreme values, and better represents the group of values.

The leak is abnormally high if the 95th leakage percentile is >24 L/min (when using a nasal mask) or if the 95th leakage percentile is >36 L/min (when using an oronasal mask), and/or the median leak is high. For advanced graphic data, the leak threshold setting is indicated by a red line at ResScan™ software (which shows the unintentional leak limit set to 24 L/min). This leak cutoff cannot be changed in the ResScan program or in the AirView remote monitoring system, even if the patient is using an oronasal mask.

It is important to note that significant leakage may impact the accuracy of PAP measurements. For example, in the presence of high unintentional leak (> 0.5 L/s or 30 L/min) it is not uncommon to observe the system algorithm pointing to unknown apnea events (apneas that cannot be defined because it occurs in the presence of large leakage).

Of course, the increase in unintentional leaks could be due to an improperly adjusted humidification chamber or damaged CPAP tubing. However, air leakage is usually due to the opening of the mouth, a poor fit of the mask, or the two causes together. The assessment of the respiratory flow curve, together with the leak chart, provides pertinent information for the diagnosis of unintentional leakage.

Normally, when air leakage occurs through the mouth, the expiratory curve is "amputated" (a sign of palatal prolapse). Interestingly, opening the mouth, even with the amputation of the exhalation curve, does not always result in an increase in unintentional leakage (Fig. 5.18).

According to some researchers, this phenomenon occurs because some patients open their mouths, but maintain a partial seal of the upper airway through the soft palate and base of the tongue [30, 31].

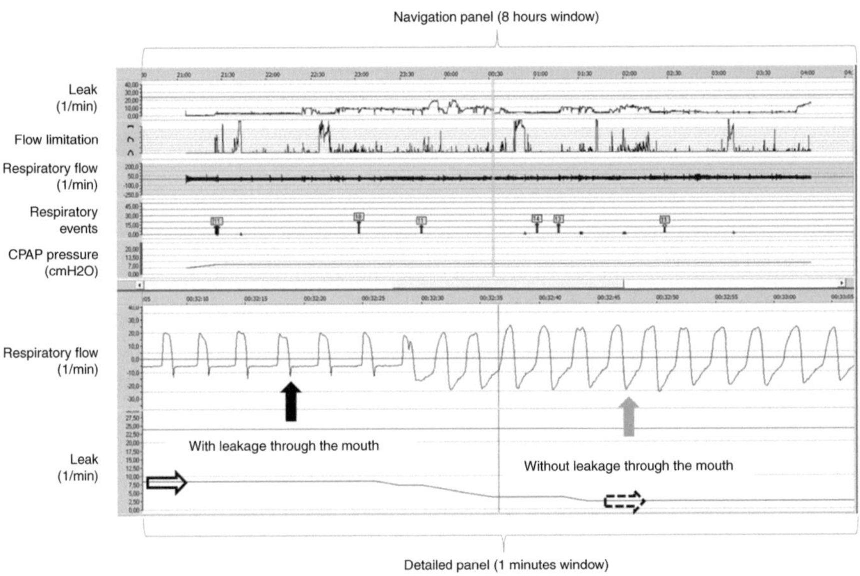

Fig. 5.18 In this figure, the black arrow shows the expiratory flow curve amputation. Notice that the leakage has also increased (open arrow). Next, we checked that the patient had closed his mouth, and the exhalation curve had improved (gray arrow). A concomitant reduction in leakage (dashed arrow) can also be observed. (Source: author's collection)

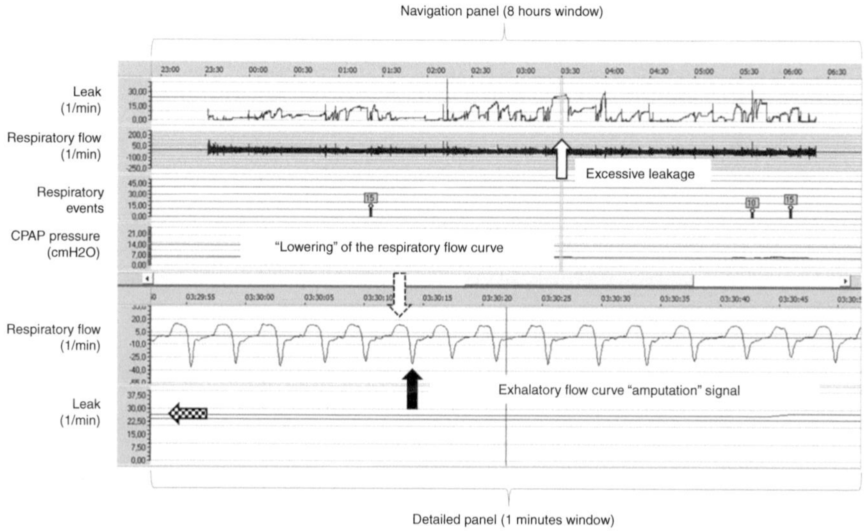

Fig. 5.19 In this illustration, the black arrow indicates the amputation of the expiratory flow curve. At the same time, one can observe the decrease in the amplitude of the inspiratory flow curve (dashed arrow). Both phenomena can indicate a leak of air through the mouth and improper fit of the mask, respectively. Leakage is over the limit of 24 L/min (check arrows and open arrows). Here, the patient is wearing a nose mask. (Source: author's collection)

When the increase in unintentional leakage occurs through the mask, it is possible to observe a decrease in the amplitude of the inspiratory flow curve, which is below what we expect for normal breathing (amplitude of the inspiratory flow curve around 20 L/min). When this amplitude is reduced, and the exhalation flow curve is amputated, it is very likely that the leak is occurring through the mouth and due to an inadequate mask adjustment (Fig. 5.19).

5.13 Palatal Prolapse

In patients with OSA, upper airway obstruction is caused by collapse in one or more sites of the pharynx during sleep (palate, tongue base, side walls, and epiglottis). Studies show that, in some individuals, the soft palate and uvula prolapsed toward the velopharynx during expiration [3]. In these cases, there is substantial pharyngeal narrowing/vibration and occasional redirection of expiratory flow out of the mouth (unidirectional airflow, i.e., inspiration through the nose and expiration through the mouth). Typically, during the assessment of the respiratory flow curve, the limitation of the expiratory flow curve can be observed (Fig. 5.20).

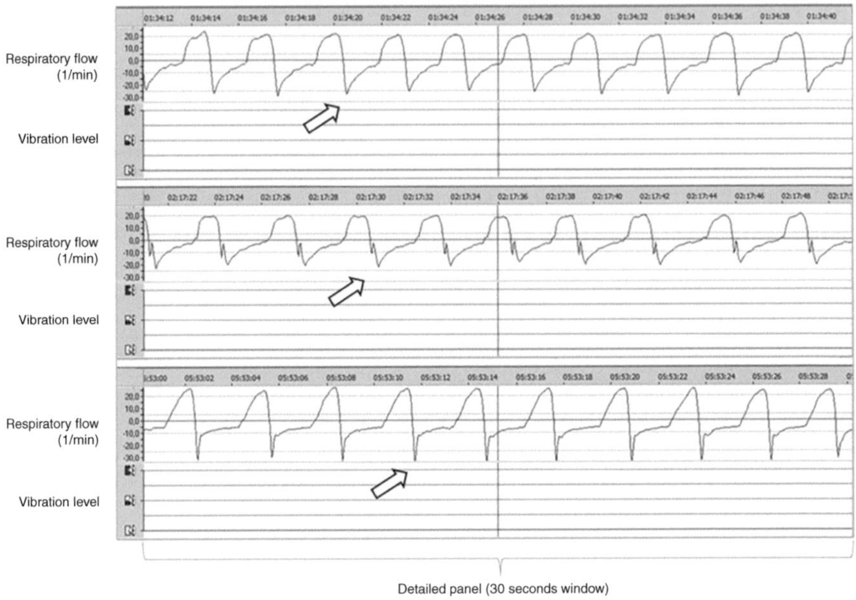

Fig. 5.20 In these examples, extracted from a single patient in the same night of positive airway pressure use, it is possible to observe that the expiratory flow curve progresses from a normal pattern to an important expiratory flow restriction (highlighted by white arrows from the upper panel to the lower panel, respectively), indicative of palatal prolapse. (Source: author's collection)

5.14 Epiglottic Collapse

In a considerable number of cases, the pattern of upper airway obstruction may be different during awakening and sleep. Drug-induced sleep endoscopy (DISE) visualizes the upper airways and has been performed many times, primarily for differential diagnostics. One of the most significant DISE findings was the collapse of the epiglottis [32].

DISE studies have shown that epiglottic collapse occurs more frequently than previously described. In fact, some studies have reported that up to 30% of patients have complete collapse of epiglottis [4]. This finding is critical because the CPAP, often considered the first-line treatment for OSA, can worsen epiglottic collapse due to associated anatomical features [32].

However, the invasive and expensive nature of DISE makes routine assessment with this instrument difficult. In addition, studies have shown that individuals with OSA have well-defined and reproducible intra-respiratory airflow characteristics during sleep. And that there is a link between reduced airflow associated with increased inspiratory effort and the presence of epiglottic collapse in the

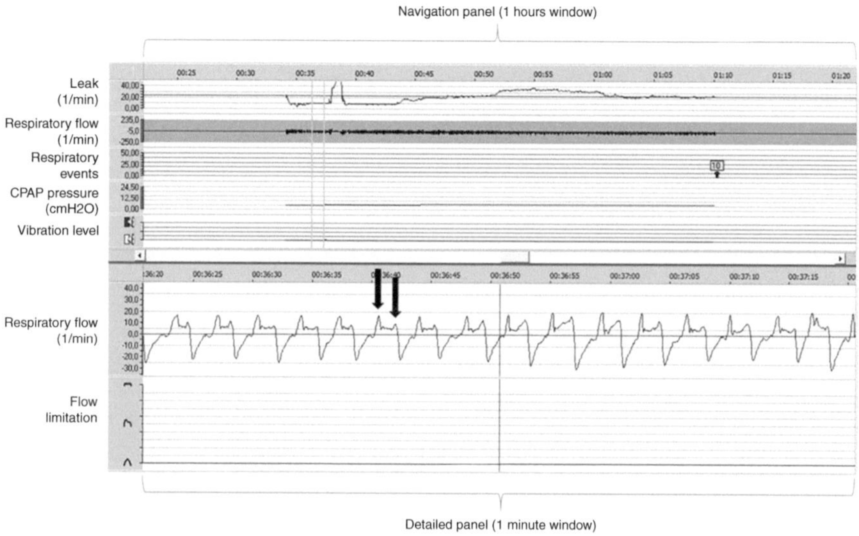

Fig. 5.21 In this respiratory flow curve example, extracted from ResMed's ResScan system, we can see in the detailed panel that the inspiratory flow curve shows two distinct effort movements in the same inspiratory phase of the respiratory cycle (highlighted by black arrows). Studies show that this would be the inspiratory flow curve pattern observed in patients with epiglottis collapse [4]. (Source: author's collection)

OSA. Furthermore, those studies suggested that rapid changes in inspiratory airflow within the same respiratory movement would be the visual marker for the recognition of epiglottic collapse [4]. Thus, the assessment of the respiratory flow curve becomes a powerful and low-cost tool for assessing epiglottic collapse (Fig. 5.21).

5.15 Equipment Turns On and Off Several Times During Sleep

In Fig. 5.22, we can see in the pressure curve, in the navigation window, that the CPAP equipment turns on and off several times during the night. This is not a malfunction of the apparatus. In that case, the device's SmartStart™ function is active. With this feature, the device turns on automatically when the patient starts breathing the mask and turns off automatically when the patient takes the mask off. However, in the event of a large unintentional leak, the equipment sensor may interpret that the interface has been removed and, therefore, automatically shuts off.

At the same Fig. 5.22, after being turned off (and then without any more excessive leakage at this moment), the equipment immediately detects the patient's

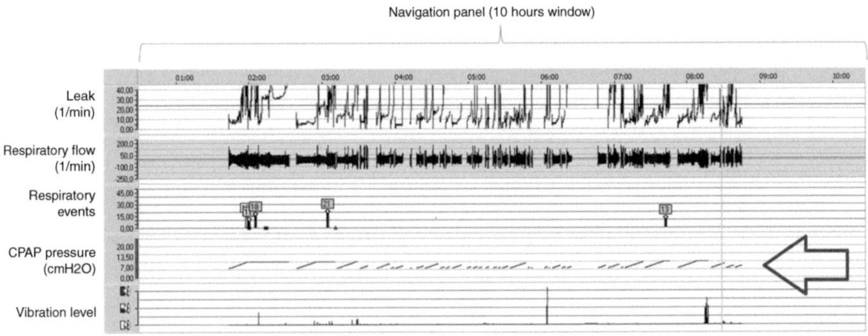

Fig. 5.22 In this figure, the open arrow shows the positive airway pressure (which has been adjusted in fixed mode). Note that the appliance turns on and off several times during the night because of excessive leaks. The auto on-off function is active. With no airflow (and no leakage after shutdown), the equipment recognizes the patient's respiratory flow again and turns on (and turns on and off continuously throughout the night). (Source: author's collection)

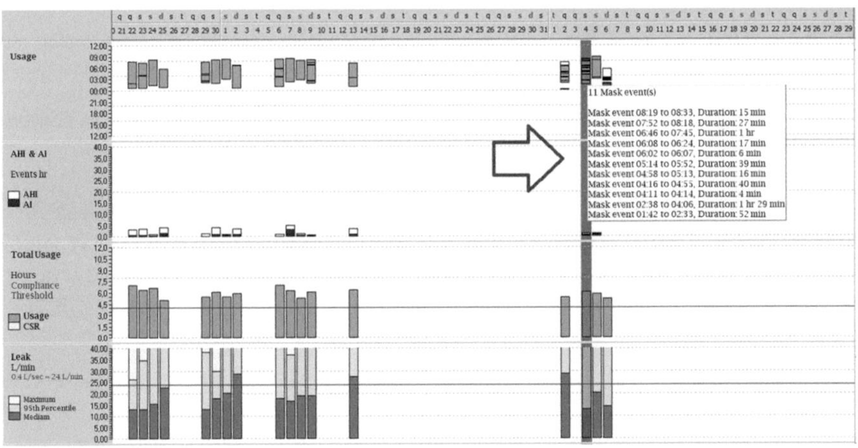

Fig. 5.23 On the same night presented in Fig. 5.22, when accessing the mask event window, there are many events (understood by the system as several mask "removal and placement" during sleep). (Source: author's collection)

breathing pattern again and turns it back on, to then turn itself off due to excessive leakage, in a countless cycle. In the summary graphic data window (Fig. 5.23), when we position the cursor over the utilization bar, a window opens and shows the large number of mask events that occurred during the night. Then changing the interface might solve the problem.

5.16 Unknown Apneas

As previously mentioned, in the presence of high involuntary leak (> 0.5 L/s or 30 L/min) it is not uncommon to observe the system algorithm pointing to unknown apnea events (apneas that cannot be defined because they occur in the presence of high leak).

Notice in the statistical report presented in Fig. 5.24 that unintentional leak is excessively high at the 95th percentile (it is also high at the median), and that the residual apnea index is also high, mainly due to unknown respiratory events.

In the detailed graphical evaluation (Fig. 5.25) at the same night, unknown apneas are concentrated in the period when the leak is so high that the upper graphical limit does not appear in the data window. It is also possible to observe that the respiratory flow curve loses its characteristics and appears as an isometric tracing, due to the failure of the system to recognize the respiratory pattern in the presence of excessive leak.

Statistics

Date (report period)	**Device**: (model)	(S/N: --------------------)
Device Settings		
Therapy Mode: **CPAP**	EPR: **RAMP ONLY**	EPR Level: **3.0 cmH2O**
EPR Enable: **ON**	EPR Patient Enable: **ON**	Ramp Enable: **ON**
Ramp Time: **5.0 Minutes**	ESSentials: **ON**	Response: **STANDARD**
Pressure: **10.6 cmH2O**		
Leak - L/min		
Median: **30.0**	95th Percentile: **79.2**	Maximum: **91.2**
Respiratory Indices - events/hr		
Apnea Index: **25.0**	Hypopnea Index: **0.6**	AHI: **25.6**
Obstructive: **4.3**	Central: **0.1**	Unknown: **20.6**
RERA Index: **0.4**	% Time in CSR: **0.0**	
Total Usage		
Used Days >= 4 hrs : **1**	Used Days < 4 hrs : **0**	% Used Days >= 4 hrs : **100**
Days not used: **0**	Total days: **1**	Total hours used: **9: 46**
Median daily usage: **9:46**	Average daily usage: **9:46**	

Fig. 5.24 In this example statistical report, the unintentional leakage in the 95th percentile is 79.2 L/min (open arrow). This specific device supports a leak of 24 L/min (wearing a nasal mask) or 36 L/min (wearing an oronasal mask), without motor overload to maintain the therapeutic pressure. Also note that the residual apnea (closed arrow) is elevated (25.6 events per hour), mainly due to the unknown apnea (20.6 events per hour). (Source: author's collection)

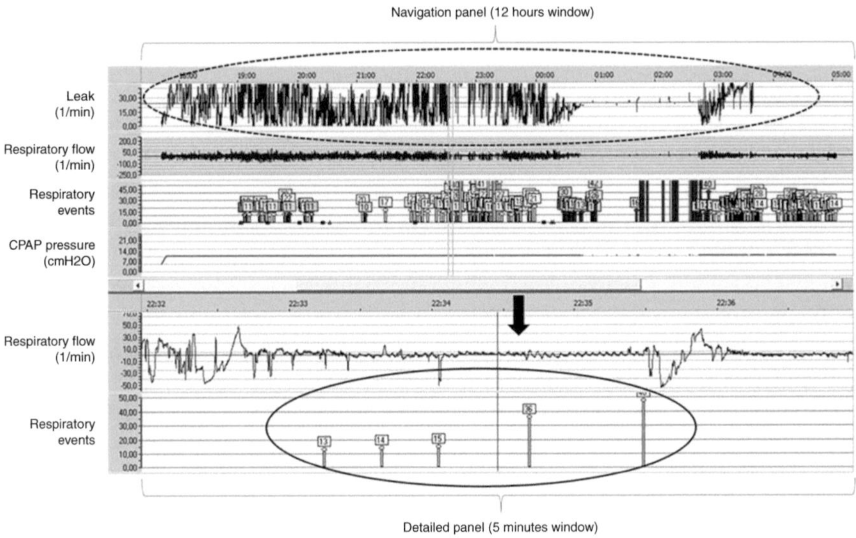

Fig. 5.25 In the detailed graphical evaluation of statistical data presented in Fig. 5.24, unknown apneas (closed circle) are detected in the period when the leak is so high that the upper graphical limit does not appear in the data window. It is also possible to observe that the respiratory flow curve loses its characteristics and appears as an isometric tracing (closed arrow), due to the failure of the system to recognize the respiratory pattern when there is excessive leak. (Source: author's collection)

5.17 Sighs

Normal respiration in humans includes breaths whose tidal volume is significantly above average. These deep breaths, called sighs, are considered an important part of normal breathing. It is well known that pulmonary compliance and functional residual capacity increase after a sigh, and this may be the result of the opening of collapsed alveoli [33]. The frequency of sighs can be altered by hypoxemia, hypercapnia, several drugs, skin stimuli, and behavioral factors. All these factors bear testimony to the complexity of the regulation of sighs. Sleep is associated with significant changes in ventilatory control and the inhibition of numerous somatic and autonomous reflexes, which may influence the onset of sighs. Sighs typically occur during all stages of sleep, including REM sleep. Light sleep can have a strong association with arousals [33]. Also, sighs may be associated with an increased risk of disordered respiratory rhythm (episodes of apnea, hypoventilation, or slowing of frequency after a sigh), depending on the phenotype patient characteristic (high loop gain or low loop gain).

There are patients who frequently sigh throughout the night and do not necessarily have altered breathing in response to sigh hyperventilation (Fig. 5.26). Interestingly, sighs can be easily detected when assessing the respiratory flow curve (extracted from the positive pressure device).

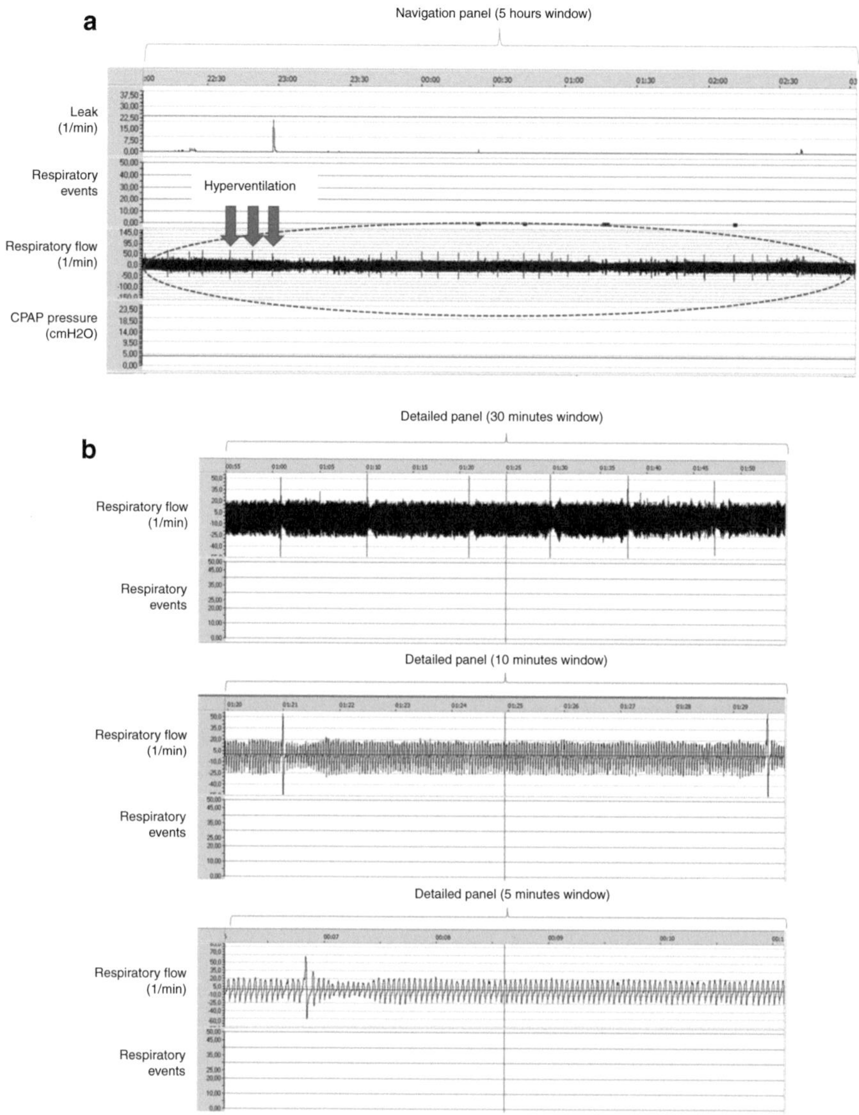

Fig. 5.26 Closed arrows highlighted the sigh at sleep (**a**). The increase in the amplitude of the respiratory flow curve can be easily detected throughout the night. In (**b**), the morphology of the respiratory flow curve when the sigh appears is highlighted in 30-, 10-, and 5-min windows. (Source: author's collection)

5.18 Catathrenia or Artifact at Exhalation Flow Curve

Also known as a sleep-related groan, in the third edition of the International Classification of Sleep Disorders, catathrenia is part of the sleep-related breathing disorders section [14, 34]. It appears to be associated with prolonged expiration, usually during REM sleep (although some studies have documented catathrenia during NREM sleep). Normally, in case of catathrenia, deep inspiration is followed by prolonged exhalation and monotonous vocalization such as moaning. The problem is generally reported by family members or relatives of the affected person. Catathrenia is rare and occurs more among males. Its cause is still unknown [35]. Multiple episodes can occur throughout the night and often in clusters of events. The long-term consequences are unknown, but the disorder is primarily a social problem for those experiencing it. Episodes of catathrenia are not associated with sleep talking or body movements, and cannot be considered as expiratory snoring (catathrenia is laryngeal, whereas snoring is guttural) [34]. Neither are they associated with psychiatric problems [34]. Recently, catathrenia has been reported in patients using sodium oxybate to treat narcolepsy with cataplexy [36]. The clinical significance of this finding is still unclear. There is little research on catathrenia, but it is associated with daytime fatigue, lack of sleep, anxiety, and social discomfort. It is believed that it may respond well to the use of CPAP, with low therapeutic pressures.

Catathrenia is not a common finding when assessing respiratory flow curves. At the PSG it is similar in appearance to a central apnea (Fig. 5.27) [36–38]. It may be difficult to identify a catathrenia episode when analyzing the respiratory flow curve, as there is no sound recording at the positive airway pressure device. However, at the respiratory flow curve analysis, a central respiratory event that presents a "snoring" data (vibration level) since the beginning, could be an indication of groan (since in central apnea the collapse of the upper airway usually does not occur). But we should be aware that a subsequent vibratory signal in a central breathing event could, on the other hand, suggest a mixed apnea (possibly with a partial upper airway opening at the second section of the respiratory event).

In our routine of respiratory flow curve analysis, changes in the exhalation flow curve, if they are not caused by palatal prolapse as mentioned earlier in this chapter, are likely due to other causes such as secretions, anatomical changes in the UA, or cardiac pulse artifact (Fig. 5.28).

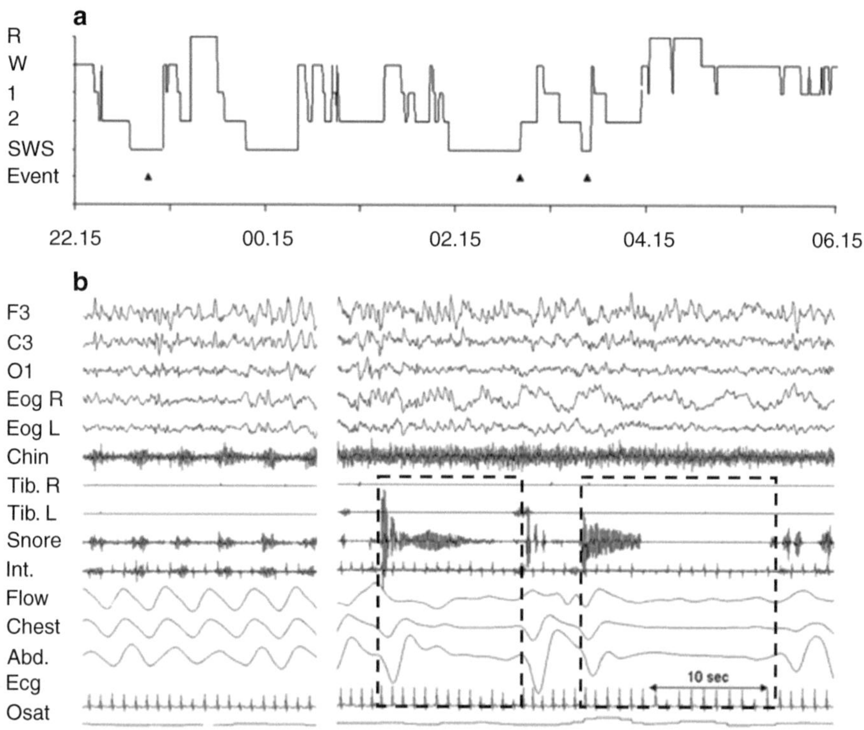

Fig. 5.27 Simple snoring (Panel **b** left) and catathrenia (Panel **b** right, dashed squares) in a 41-year-old male patient treated with sodium oxybate (SO). (**a**) Polysomnographic histogram. Triangles indicate the episodes of recurrent catathrenia. *R* REM sleep, *W* wakefulness, 1 stage: 1 NREM sleep, 2 stage: 2 NREM sleep, SWS: slow wave sleep, Event: catathrenia. (**b**) F3, C3, O: electroencephalogram; Eog R, Eog L right and left: electrooculogram; Chin: submentalis muscle electromyogram; Tib. R, Tib. L right and left: tibialis anterior muscle electromyogram; Snore microphone; Int. intercostalis: muscle electromyogram; Flow: oral respirogram; Chest: thoracic respirogram; Abd: abdominal respirogram; Ecg: electrocardiogram; Osat: oxygen saturation. Polysomnographic traces: on the left, simple inspiratory snoring during NREM sleep; on the right, clusters of catathrenia resembling central apnea during NREM sleep, differentiated by the presence of moaning. The catathrenic breathing pattern is characterized by a deep inspiration followed by a prolonged expiration without appreciable oxygen desaturation. An EEG arousal marks the beginning of the catathrenic cluster. (Source: Poli F et al. Sleep Breath, 2012. With permission. In our routine of respiratory flow curve analysis, changes in the exhalation flow curve, if they are not caused by palatal prolapse as mentioned earlier in this chapter, are likely due to other causes such as secretions, anatomical changes in the UA, or cardiac pulse artifact (Fig. 5.28))

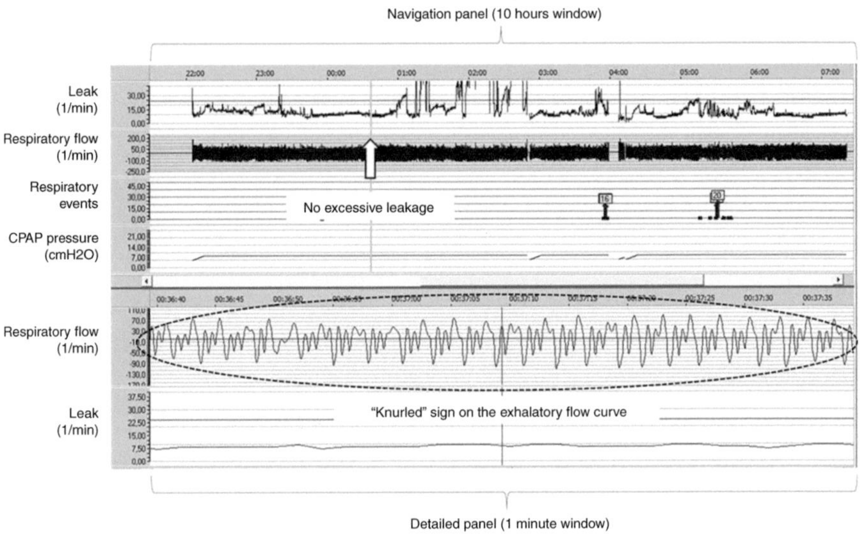

Fig. 5.28 In this illustration, the dashed circle highlights examples of a respiratory flow curve, with a significant change in the expiration tracing, where there is even difficulty in distinguishing between the inspiratory and expiratory phases. Most likely a carotid pulse artifact. (Source: author's collection)

5.19 Oximetry Module

The oximetry module is a highly functional piece of equipment that easily links the XPOD oximeter to the positive airway pressure system. The module is user-friendly and easy to install. The oximeter works to record oxygen saturation levels and heart rate, which can be evaluated concomitantly with the graphic information of the respiratory flow curve during sleep and with the other high-resolution graphic information provided by the ResScan™ system (Fig. 5.29).

Oximetry has been very useful in assessing oxygen saturation in patients who are treating sleep-related breathing disorders with PAP therapy, when an associated ventilatory disorder is suspected (i.e., hypoventilation due to obesity or chronic obstructive pulmonary disease).

In the example provided in Fig. 5.30, a severe OSA patient was submitted to oximetry evaluation concomitantly with the use of positive pressure device (fixed pressure of 11 cmH_2O), at air room. The same patient was later submitted to oximetry evaluation concomitantly with the use of bi-level positive pressure device (inspiratory pressure of 15 cmH_2O and an expiratory pressure of 11 cmH_2O), at air room (Fig. 5.31).

Note that both positive airway pressure modes are effective for improving OSA, but the bilevel device was better for improving oxygenation.

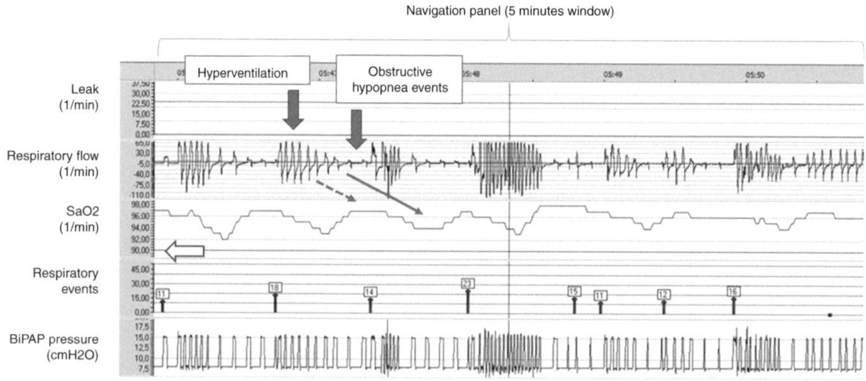

Fig. 5.29 In this figure, on the respiratory flow curve, one can notice a periodic breathing pattern (when using a bi-level positive airway device). On the SaO_2 window, a desaturation is observed after a hypopnea (straight line), and an improved oxygen saturation is observed immediately after a hyperventilation event (dashed line). Note that even within a periodic respiratory pattern, there was no oxygen desaturation below 90% (open arrow indicates 90% saturation threshold). (Source: author's collection)

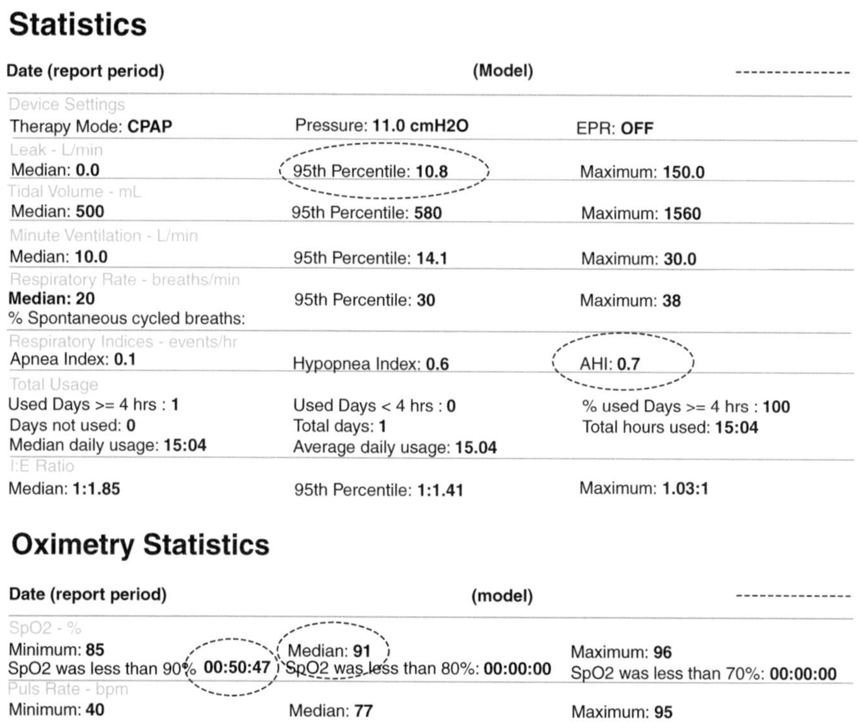

Statistics

Date (report period)	(Model)	---------------
Device Settings		
Therapy Mode: **CPAP**	Pressure: **11.0 cmH2O**	EPR: **OFF**
Leak - L/min		
Median: **0.0**	95th Percentile: **10.8**	Maximum: **150.0**
Tidal Volume - mL		
Median: **500**	95th Percentile: **580**	Maximum: **1560**
Minute Ventilation - L/min		
Median: **10.0**	95th Percentile: **14.1**	Maximum: **30.0**
Respiratory Rate - breaths/min		
Median: 20 % Spontaneous cycled breaths:	95th Percentile: **30**	Maximum: **38**
Respiratory Indices - events/hr		
Apnea Index: **0.1**	Hypopnea Index: **0.6**	AHI: **0.7**
Total Usage		
Used Days >= 4 hrs : **1** Days not used: **0** Median daily usage: **15:04**	Used Days < 4 hrs : **0** Total days: **1** Average daily usage: **15.04**	% used Days >= 4 hrs : **100** Total hours used: **15:04**
I:E Ratio		
Median: **1:1.85**	95th Percentile: **1:1.41**	Maximum: **1.03:1**

Oximetry Statistics

Date (report period)	(model)	---------------
SpO2 - %		
Minimum: **85** SpO2 was less than 90% **00:50:47**	Median: **91** SpO2 was less than 80%: **00:00:00**	Maximum: **96** SpO2 was less than 70%: **00:00:00**
Puls Rate - bpm		
Minimum: **40**	Median: **77**	Maximum: **95**

Fig. 5.30 In this statistical report, the patient is using a positive airway pressure device in a fixed positive airway pressure mode (pressure of 11.0 cmH_2O). The leakage is controlled, as well as the residual apnea index (0.7 events per hour of sleep). Median oxygen saturation (SaO_2) was 89%, but the patient remained at SaO_2 below 90% for over 50 min. (Source: author's collection)

Statistics

Date (report period)	(Model)	---------------
Device Settings		
Therapy Mode: **SPONT**	Expiration Pressure: **11.0 cmH2O**	Inspiration Pressure: **15.0 cmH2O**
Leak - L/min		
Median: **0.0**	95th Percentile: **24.0**	Maximum: **148.8**
Tidal Volume - mL		
Median: **560**	95th Percentile: **640**	Maximum: **1320**
Minute Ventilation - L/min		
Median: **11.3**	95th Percentile: **16.5**	Maximum: **29.8**
Respiratory Rate - breaths/min		
Median: 20	95th Percentile: **28**	Maximum: **38**
% Spontaneous cycled breaths: **99**		
Respiratory Indices - events/hr		
Apnea Index: **0.6**	Hypopnea Index: **0.0**	AHI: **0.6**
Total Usage		
Used Days >= 4 hrs : **1**	Used Days < 4 hrs : **0**	% used Days >= 4 hrs : **100**
Days not used: **0**	Total days: **1**	Total hours used: **13:05**
Median daily usage: **13:05**	Average daily usage: **13.05**	
I:E Ratio		
Median: **1:1.92**	95th Percentile: **1:1.56**	Maximum: **1:1.33**

Oximetry Statistics

Date (report period)	(model)	---------------
SpO2 - %		
Minimum: **89**	Median: **93**	Maximum: **97**
SpO2 was less than 90% **00:00:40**	SpO2 was less than 80%: **00:00:00**	SpO2 was less than 70%: **00:00:00**
Puls Rate - bpm		
Minimum: **62**	Median: **71**	Maximum: **91**

Fig. 5.31 In this statistical report, the patient is using a bilevel positive airway pressure device (inspiratory pressure of 15 cmH_2O and expiratory pressure of 11 cmH_2O). The leakage is controlled, as well as the residual apnea index (0.6 events per hour of sleep). Median oxygen saturation (SaO_2) was 93%, and the patient stayed with SaO_2 under 90% for only 40 s. (Source: author's collection)

When it is impossible to use the oximetry module, and an associated ventilatory disorder is suspected, there are other devices that also can help a lot in ventilatory assessment at home, such as the wireless high-resolution oximeter [39].

5.20 Isometric Airway Flow Curve Trace

When unknown apneas were addressed in this chapter, it was commented on the possibility that the pattern of the respiratory flow curve was not adequately defined by the equipment algorithm, in the presence of high unintentional leak. In this occurrence, the respiratory flow curve is typically presented as an isometric waveform. However, this same isometric pattern can be seen without excessive leakage. Therefore, the problem lies in determining what might interfere with the detection

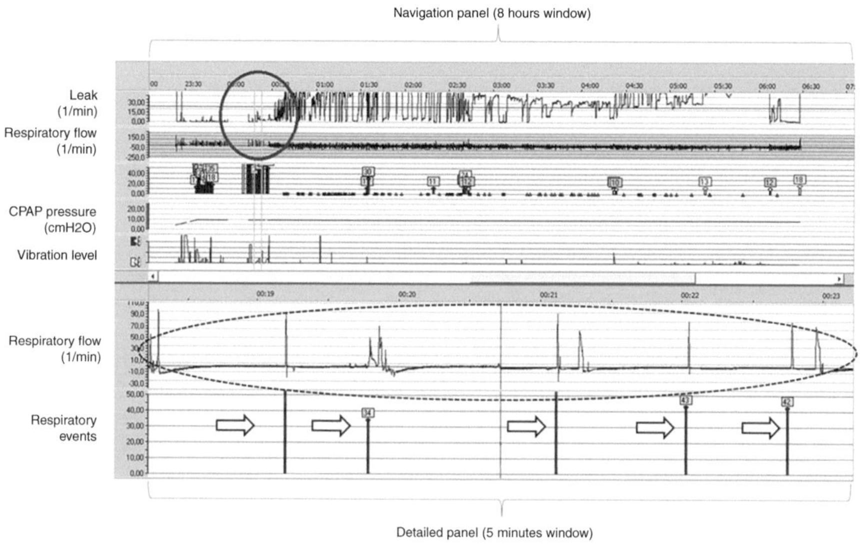

Fig. 5.32 Isometric waveform of the respiratory flow curve (dashed circle), due to interrupted flow in a hollow tubular mask, pressing the side of the mask with the arm, while sleeping. Note that excessive air leakage (closed circle) does not occur. (Source: author's collection)

of the appropriate respiratory flow curve. This is usually due to the fact that the mask is incorrectly positioned on the patient's face, or poorly assembled (like inverted cushions, for example). We have already observed this same problem due to the interruption of flow in hollow-frame tubing masks, when the patient is sleeping on his side but has the habit of pressing his arm over his head, interrupting adequate airflow through the mask sides (Fig. 5.32).

5.21 Further Reading

This is an unprecedented book and so far, there is no written material that gathers in a single place detailed information of respiratory flow curves analysis, extracted from positive airway pressure devices to the treatment of sleep breathing disorders.

A vast bibliography was presented in this chapter and the reading of this material will help in consolidating the understanding of the advanced graphical examples (mainly the respiratory flow curves during sleep). However, knowledge of respiratory physiology and pathophysiology, as well as sleep fundamentals, is also essential. To achieve this, we recommend reading books: West JB. Respiratory Physiology: The essentials [40], West's Pulmonary Pathophysiology: The Essentials [41] and Principles and Practice of Sleep Medicine (Meir Kryger TR) [42].

References

1. Gugger M, Mathis J, Bassetti C. Accuracy of an intelligent CPAP machine with in-built diagnostic abilities in detecting apnoeas: a comparison with polysomnography. Thorax. 1995;50(11):1199–201. https://doi.org/10.1136/thx.50.11.1199.
2. Azarbarzin A, Sands SA, Taranto-Montemurro L, Oliveira Marques MD, Genta PR, Edwards BA, et al. Estimation of pharyngeal collapsibility during sleep by peak inspiratory airflow. Sleep. 2017;40(1):zsw005. https://doi.org/10.1093/sleep/zsw005.
3. Azarbarzin A, Sands SA, Marques M, Genta PR, Taranto-Montemurro L, Messineo L, et al. Palatal prolapse as a signature of expiratory flow limitation and inspiratory palatal collapse in patients with obstructive sleep apnoea. Eur Respir J. 2018;51(2):1701419. https://doi.org/10.1183/13993003.01419-2017.
4. Azarbarzin A, Marques M, Sands SA, Op de Beeck S, Genta PR, Taranto-Montemurro L, et al. Predicting epiglottic collapse in patients with obstructive sleep apnoea. Eur Respir J. 2017;50(3):1700345. https://doi.org/10.1183/13993003.00345-2017.
5. Ayappa I, Norman RG, Whiting D, Tsai AH, Anderson F, Donnely E, et al. Irregular respiration as a marker of wakefulness during titration of CPAP. Sleep. 2009;32(1):99–104.
6. Sands SA, Owens RL. Congestive heart failure and central sleep apnea. Sleep Med Clin. 2016;11(1):127–42. https://doi.org/10.1016/j.jsmc.2015.10.003.
7. Weinreich G, Armitstead J, Teschler H. Pattern recognition of obstructive sleep apnoea and Cheyne-stokes respiration. Physiol Meas. 2008;29(8):869–78. https://doi.org/10.1088/0967-3334/29/8/002.
8. Stevens D, Martins RT, Mukherjee S, Vakulin A. Post-stroke sleep-disordered breathing-pathophysiology and therapy options. Front Surg. 2018;5:9. https://doi.org/10.3389/fsurg.2018.00009.
9. Neill AM, Angus SM, Sajkov D, McEvoy RD. Effects of sleep posture on upper airway stability in patients with obstructive sleep apnea. Am J Respir Crit Care Med. 1997;155(1):199–204. https://doi.org/10.1164/ajrccm.155.1.9001312.
10. Marques M, Genta PR, Sands SA, Azarbazin A, de Melo C, Taranto-Montemurro L, et al. Effect of sleeping position on upper airway patency in obstructive sleep apnea is determined by the pharyngeal structure causing collapse. Sleep. 2017;40(3):zsx005. https://doi.org/10.1093/sleep/zsx005.
11. Javaheri S, Barbe F, Campos-Rodriguez F, Dempsey JA, Khayat R, Malhotra A, et al. Sleep apnea: types, mechanisms, and clinical cardiovascular consequences. J Am Coll Cardiol. 2017;69(7):841–58. https://doi.org/10.1016/j.jacc.2016.11.069.
12. Terziyski K, Draganova A. Central sleep apnea with Cheyne-stokes breathing in heart failure—from research to clinical practice and beyond. Adv Exp Med Biol. 2018;1067:327–51. https://doi.org/10.1007/5584_2018_146.
13. White LH, Bradley TD. Role of nocturnal rostral fluid shift in the pathogenesis of obstructive and central sleep apnoea. J Physiol. 2013;591(5):1179–93. https://doi.org/10.1113/jphysiol.2012.245159.
14. Barry R, Albertario CL. The AASM manual for the scoring of sleep and associates events: rules, terminology and technical specifications. Version 2.5. Darien, IL: American Academy of Sleep Medicine; 2018.
15. Burgess KR, Lucas SJ, Shepherd K, Dawson A, Swart M, Thomas KN, et al. Worsening of central sleep apnea at high altitude—a role for cerebrovascular function. J Appl Physiol. 2013;114(8):1021–8. https://doi.org/10.1152/japplphysiol.01462.2012.
16. Parra O, Arboix A, Bechich S, García-Eroles L, Montserrat JM, López JA, et al. Time course of sleep-related breathing disorders in first-ever stroke or transient ischemic attack. Am J Respir Crit Care Med. 2000;161(2 Pt 1):375–80. https://doi.org/10.1164/ajrccm.161.2.9903139.
17. Gaig C, Iranzo A. Sleep-disordered breathing in neurodegenerative diseases. Curr Neurol Neurosci Rep. 2012;12(2):205–17. https://doi.org/10.1007/s11910-011-0248-1.

18. Issa FG, Sullivan CE. Reversal of central sleep apnea using nasal CPAP. Chest. 1986;90(2):165–71. https://doi.org/10.1378/chest.90.2.165.
19. Liu P, Chen Q, Yuan F, Zhang Q, Zhang X, Xue C, et al. Clinical predictors of mixed apneas in patients with obstructive sleep apnea (OSA). Nat Sci Sleep. 2022;14:373–80. https://doi.org/10.2147/NSS.S351946.
20. Zhang J, Wang L, Guo HJ, Wang Y, Cao J, Chen BY. Treatment-emergent central sleep apnea: a unique sleep-disordered breathing. Chin Med J. 2020;133(22):2721–30. https://doi.org/10.1097/CM9.0000000000001125.
21. Berry RB, Brooks R, Gamaldo C, Harding SM, Lloyd RM, Quan SF, et al. AASM scoring manual updates for 2017 (version 2.4). J Clin Sleep Med. 2017;13(5):665–6. https://doi.org/10.5664/jcsm.6576.
22. Randerath WJ, Treml M, Priegnitz C, Stieglitz S, Hagmeyer L, Morgenstern C. Evaluation of a noninvasive algorithm for differentiation of obstructive and central hypopneas. Sleep. 2013;36(3):363–8. https://doi.org/10.5665/sleep.2450.
23. Ogna A, Tobback N, Andries D, Preisig M, Vollenweider P, Waeber G, et al. Prevalence and clinical significance of respiratory effort-related arousals in the general population. J Clin Sleep Med. 2018;14(8):1339–45. https://doi.org/10.5664/jcsm.7268.
24. Berry RB, Quan SF, Abreu AR, Bibbs ML, DelRosso L, Harding SM, et al. The AASM manual for the scoring of sleep and associated events: rules, terminology and technical specifications. Darien, IL: American Academy of Sleep Medicine; 2020.
25. Ayappa I, Norman RG, Suryadevara M, Rapoport DM. Comparison of limited monitoring using a nasal-cannula flow signal to full polysomnography in sleep-disordered breathing. Sleep. 2004;27(6):1171–9. https://doi.org/10.1093/sleep/27.6.1171.
26. Oudiette D, Dodet P, Ledard N, Artru E, Rachidi I, Similowski T, et al. REM sleep respiratory behaviours mental content in narcoleptic lucid dreamers. Sci Rep. 2018;8(1):2636. https://doi.org/10.1038/s41598-018-21067-9.
27. Kubin L, Davies RO, Pack AI. Control of upper airway Motoneurons during REM sleep. News Physiol Sci. 1998;13:91–7. https://doi.org/10.1152/physiologyonline.1998.13.2.91.
28. Edwards BA, O'Driscoll DM, Ali A, Jordan AS, Trinder J, Malhotra A. Aging and sleep: physiology and pathophysiology. Semin Respir Crit Care Med. 2010;31(5):618–33. https://doi.org/10.1055/s-0030-1265902.
29. Deacon-Diaz N, Malhotra A. Inherent vs. induced loop gain abnormalities in obstructive sleep apnea. Front Neurol. 2018;9:896. https://doi.org/10.3389/fneur.2018.00896.
30. Genta PR, Sands SA, Butler JP, Loring SH, Katz ES, Demko BG, et al. Airflow shape is associated with the pharyngeal structure causing OSA. Chest. 2017;152(3):537–46. https://doi.org/10.1016/j.chest.2017.06.017.
31. Genta PR, Kaminska M, Edwards BA, Ebben MR, Krieger AC, Tamisier R, et al. The importance of mask selection on continuous positive airway pressure outcomes for obstructive sleep apnea. An official American Thoracic Society workshop report. Ann Am Thorac Soc. 2020;17(10):1177–85. https://doi.org/10.1513/AnnalsATS.202007-864ST.
32. Kim HY, Sung CM, Jang HB, Kim HC, Lim SC, Yang HC. Patients with epiglottic collapse showed less severe obstructive sleep apnea and good response to treatment other than continuous positive airway pressure: a case-control study of 224 patients. J Clin Sleep Med. 2021;17(3):413–9. https://doi.org/10.5664/jcsm.8904.
33. Perez-Padilla R, West P, Kryger MH. Sighs during sleep in adult humans. Sleep. 1983;6(3):234–43. https://doi.org/10.1093/sleep/6.3.234.
34. Alonso J, Camacho M, Chhetri DK, Guilleminault C, Zaghi S. Catathrenia (nocturnal groaning): a social media survey and state-of-the-art review. J Clin Sleep Med. 2017;13(4):613–22. https://doi.org/10.5664/jcsm.6556.
35. Rodrigues DM, Valério MP, Costa T. Catathrenia—a rare but disturbing sleep disorder. Arch Bronconeumol (Engl Ed). 2021;57(10):654. https://doi.org/10.1016/j.arbres.2021.01.022.

36. Poli F, Ricotta L, Vandi S, Franceschini C, Pizza F, Palaia V, et al. Catathrenia under sodium oxybate in narcolepsy with cataplexy. Sleep Breath. 2012;16(2):427–34. https://doi.org/10.1007/s11325-011-0520-2.
37. Petitto L, Com G, Jackson R, Richter G, Jambhekar S. Catathrenia and treatment with positive airway pressure in the pediatric population. J Clin Sleep Med. 2019;15(12):1853–7. https://doi.org/10.5664/jcsm.8100.
38. Ramar K, Olson EJ, Morgenthaler TI. Catathrenia. Sleep Med. 2008;9(4):457–9. https://doi.org/10.1016/j.sleep.2007.08.011.
39. Hasan R, Genta PR, Pinheiro GDL, Garcia ML, Scudeller PG, de Carvalho CRR, et al. Validation of an overnight wireless high-resolution oximeter for the diagnosis of obstructive sleep apnea at home. Sci Rep. 2022;12(1):15136. https://doi.org/10.1038/s41598-022-17698-8.
40. West JB. Respiratory physiology: the essentials. 9th ed. Philadelphia: Lippincott Williams Wilkins/Wolters Kluwer Business; 2012.
41. West J, Luks A. West's pulmonary pathophysiology: the essentials. 10th ed. Philadelphia: Wolters Kluwer; 2021.
42. Meir Kryger TR, William C. Dement. Principles and practice of sleep medicine. 6th ed. Amsterdam: Elsevier; 2017.

Part 2
Monitoring Positive Pressure Therapy in Sleep-Related Breathing Disorders: Advanced Analysis of Respiratory Flow Curves/Case Reports

In this section of the book are present clinical cases in which the analysis of respiratory flow curves was part of the patient's therapeutic evaluation process.

Chapter 6
Case Report: Obstructive Sleep Apnea Developed into Central Sleep Apnea After a Stroke

6.1 Patient Information

An 81-year-old male, BMI 24.5 kg/m^2, was referred for PAP therapy. Diagnostic polysomnography exhibited an apnea-hypopnea index of 48.0 respiratory events/hour (mainly obstructive respiratory events). Comorbidities: cardiomyopathy, high blood pressure, complete arthroplasty of the right hip. Initiation of PAP treatment with a fixed CPAP (11.6 cmH_2O) and an oronasal mask (patient could not adapt to a nasal mask due to excessive oral leakage and patient discomfort). Adherence to pressure therapy was a success. The patient was monitored for 285 days, with maintenance of the OSA resolution and excellent compliance scores (Fig. 6.1).

Unfortunately, after this follow-up period, the patient suffered a stroke while asleep and remained hospitalized in the intensive care unit for 18 days. We were not able to observe the flow curve of the night in which the patient suffered from the stroke, as the patient's equipment model did not allow the visualization of advanced data after a brief period of time. However, by looking at the data in the statistical reports, we verified a sudden change in the patient's breathing, with many residual respiratory events that night (Fig. 6.2).

When he returned to his home, the assessment of the CPAP data revealed the persistence of residual breathing events above what is considered normal (Fig. 6.3). In the respiratory flow curve evaluation, residual obstructive respiratory events (but with characteristics of central respiratory events) were observed (Fig. 6.4).

V. S. Piccin, *Monitoring Positive Pressure Therapy in Sleep-Related Breathing Disorders*, https://doi.org/10.1007/978-3-031-50292-7_6

Statistics

Date (report period)	Device (Model)	(S/N: -----------)
Device Settings		
Therapy Mode: **CPAP**	EPR: **FULL TIME**	EPR Level: **2.0 cmH2O**
EPR Enable: **ON**	EPR Patient Enable: **ON**	Ramp Enable: **ON**
Ramp Time: **20.0 Minutes**	Essentials: **ON**	Response: **STANDARD**
Pressure: **11.6 cmH2O**		
Leak - L/min		
Median: **0.0**	95th Percentile: **10.8**	Maximum: **32.4**
Respiratory Indices - events/hr		
Apnea Index: **1.2**	Hypopnea Index: **1.1**	AHI: **2.3**
Obstructive: **0.7**	Central: **0.1**	Unknown: **0.0**
RERA Index: **0.0**	% Time in CSR: **0.0**	
Total Usage		
Used Days >= 4 hrs : **264**	Used Days < 4 hrs : **10**	% Used Days >= 4 hrs : **92**
Days not used: **11**	Total days: **285**	Total hours used: **2266:46**
Median daily usage: **8:18**	Average daily usage: **7.57**	

Fig. 6.1 The CPAP statistical report screen extracted from the equipment and visualized in the ResScan™ system. The patient's CPAP compliance is observed on that data. Compliance is often defined as the use of CPAP for an average of 4 h per night for a minimum of 70% of nights. OSA severity is defined as mild for the apnea-hypopnea index (AHI) ≥ 5 and < 15, moderate for AHI ≥ 15 and ≤ 30, and severe for AHI > 30/h. [1]. The patient's mean AHI over a 285-day period of CPAP use was 2.3 events per hour (dotted circle), indicating apnea resolution. (Source: Author's collection)

Statistics

Date (report period)	Device (Model)	(S/N: -----------)
Device Settings		
Therapy Mode: **CPAP**	EPR: **FULL TIME**	EPR Level: **2.0 cmH2O**
EPR Enable: **ON**	EPR Patient Enable: **ON**	Ramp Enable: **ON**
Ramp Time: **20.0 Minutes**	Essentials: **ON**	Response: **STANDARD**
Pressure: **11.6 cmH2O**		
Leak - L/min		
Median: **1.2**	95th Percentile: **16.8**	Maximum: **136.8**
Respiratory Indices - events/hr		
Apnea Index: **18.1**	Hypopnea Index: **1.1**	AHI: **19.2**
Obstructive: **13.1**	Central: **1.7**	Unknown: **5.2**
RERA Index: **0.0**	% Time in CSR: **0.0**	
Total Usage		
Used Days >= 4 hrs : **1**	Used Days < 4 hrs : **1**	% Used Days >= 4 hrs : **100**
Days not used: **0**	Total days: **1**	Total hours used: **6:46**
Median daily usage: **6:46**	Average daily usage: **6.46**	

Fig. 6.2 The CPAP statistical report screen extracted from the equipment and visualized in the ResScan™ system. We observe in this data the patient's CPAP statistical report overnight when he suffered a stroke. Numerous residual respiratory events (dotted circle) can also be observed in contrast to routine residual respiratory events as shown in Fig. 6.1. (Source: Author's collection)

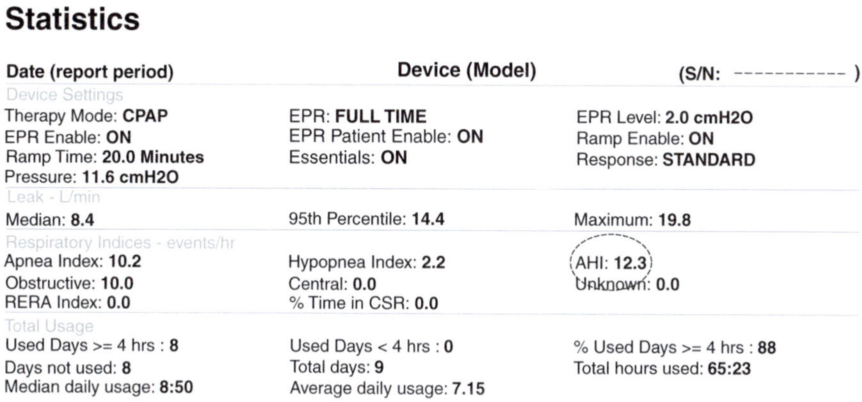

Statistics

Date (report period)	Device (Model)	(S/N: -----------)
Device Settings		
Therapy Mode: **CPAP**	EPR: **FULL TIME**	EPR Level: **2.0 cmH2O**
EPR Enable: **ON**	EPR Patient Enable: **ON**	Ramp Enable: **ON**
Ramp Time: **20.0 Minutes**	Essentials: **ON**	Response: **STANDARD**
Pressure: **11.6 cmH2O**		
Leak - L/min		
Median: **8.4**	95th Percentile: **14.4**	Maximum: **19.8**
Respiratory Indices - events/hr		
Apnea Index: **10.2**	Hypopnea Index: **2.2**	AHI: **12.3**
Obstructive: **10.0**	Central: **0.0**	Unknown: **0.0**
RERA Index: **0.0**	% Time in CSR: **0.0**	
Total Usage		
Used Days >= 4 hrs : **8**	Used Days < 4 hrs : **0**	% Used Days >= 4 hrs : **88**
Days not used: **8**	Total days: **9**	Total hours used: **65:23**
Median daily usage: **8:50**	Average daily usage: **7.15**	

Fig. 6.3 The CPAP statistical report screen extracted from the equipment and visualized in the ResScan™ system. We observe patient CPAP compliance with this data. Compliance is often defined as the use of CPAP for an average of 4 hours per night for a minimum of 70% of nights. OSA severity is defined as mild for the apnea-hypopnea index (AHI) ≥ 5 and < 15, moderate for AHI ≥ 15 and ≤ 30, and severe for AHI > 30/h. [2, 3]. The patient's mean AHI over a 9-day period of CPAP use was 12.3 events per hour (dotted circle), indicating mild apnea. (Source: Author's collection)

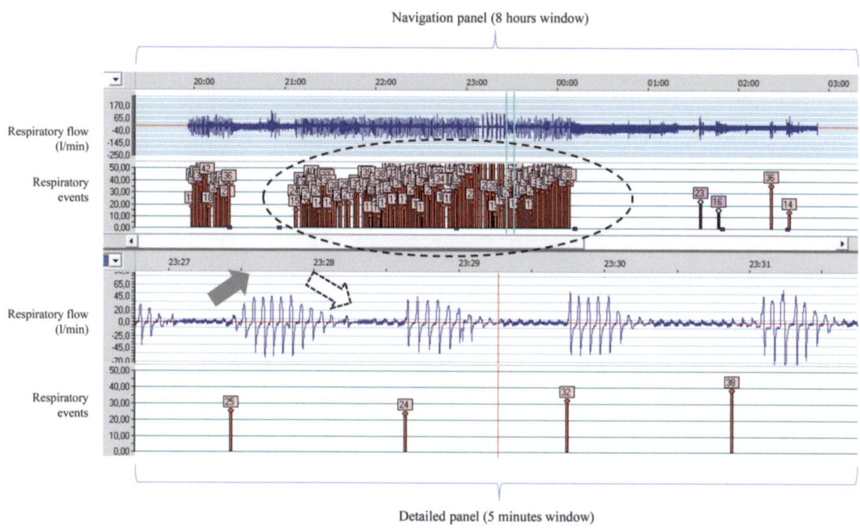

Fig. 6.4 The screen for a graphical presentation of the ResScan™ data taken from the ResMed positive pressure equipment. In the upper window, we can see numerous residual respiratory events (dotted circle), presented by the CPAP algorithm as obstructive events. At the 5-min window, we can observe a more detailed respiratory flow curve, signaling characteristics of central respiratory events, such as a progressive decrease (gray arrow) and progressive increase in the inspiratory curve (dotted arrow). (Source: Author's collection)

6.2 Therapeutic Intervention

Because the previous diagnosis of primarily obstructive respiratory events was known, it was decided to maintain pressure therapy in the fixed CPAP mode at 11.6 cmH_2O. A gradual change in the shape of the respiratory flow curve, with central apnea events been replaced by respiratory events with central hypopnea characteristics (no flattening of the inspiratory flow curve, but a decrease in amplitude of the respiratory flow curve, characteristic of a central component) can be seen in Fig. 6.5.

Moreover, in a short period of time, good control of residual IAH was observed (Table 6.1). During follow-up with the patient, we performed a small increase in therapeutic pressure to correct the limitation of the inspiratory flow curve during sleep (11.6–12.0 cmH_2O).

Surprisingly, during a subsequent follow-up visit, a residual respiratory event increased in the equipment statistic report (Fig. 6.6).

And when we observed the flow curve tracing, we found that residual respiratory events did not occur every night (Fig. 6.7) and that, when they did occur, they were consistent with the hypothesis of mixed respiratory events (Fig. 6.8).

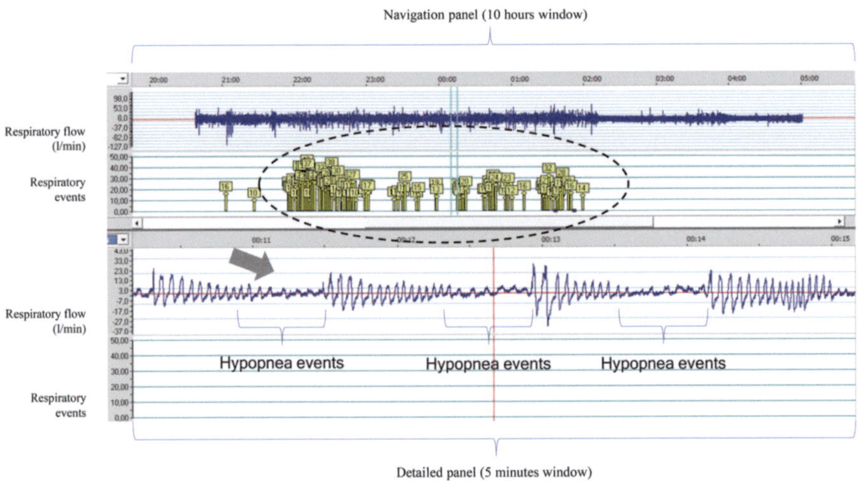

Fig. 6.5 The screen for a graphical presentation of the ResScan™ data taken from the ResMed positive pressure equipment. In the upper window, we can see numerous residual respiratory events (dotted circle), presented by the CPAP algorithm as unknown respiratory events. At the 5-min window, we can observe a more detailed respiratory flow curve, signaling characteristics of central respiratory events, such as a progressive decrease (gray arrow) on the inspiratory curve followed by hypopnea respiratory events. (Source: Author's collection)

Table 6.1 Presents the major results of the 59-day period of use of the CPAP, 1 month after the stroke. We can observe a good control of residual AHI (4.3 event/h). OSA severity is defined as mild for the apnea-hypopnea index (AHI) ≥ 5 and < 15, moderate for AHI ≥ 15 and ≤ 30, and severe for AHI > 30/h [2, 3]. (Source: Author's collection)

	59 days-period of CPAP usage
Days of use/total days (percentile of over 4 h of use per night)	55/59 (86%)
Mask	Oronasal
Pressure—cmH_2O	12.0
Average use (total number of days)—Hours	5:47
Median use (days used)—Hours	6:37
Expiratory relief	2/only ramp
95th percentile leakage—L/min	0.0
Median leakage—L/min.	0.0
Events per hour (residual AHI)	4.3
Central apnea index	0.1
Obstructive apnea index	1.6
Obstructive hypopnea index	2.7
Unknown apnea index	0.0

Statistics

Date (report period)	Device (Model)	(S/N: -----------)
Device Settings		
Therapy Mode: **CPAP**	EPR: **FULL TIME**	EPR Level: **2.0 cmH2O**
EPR Enable: **ON**	EPR Patient Enable: **ON**	Ramp Enable: **ON**
Ramp Time: **20.0 Minutes**	Essentials: **ON**	Response: **STANDARD**
Pressure: **12.0 cmH2O**		
Leak - L/min		
Median: **8.4**	95th Percentile: **3.0**	Maximum: **25.2**
Respiratory Indices - events/hr		
Apnea Index: **14.8**	Hypopnea Index: **2.1**	AHI: **16.9**
Obstructive: **13.2**	Central: **0.3**	Unknown: **0.0**
RERA Index: **0.0**	% Time in CSR: **0.0**	
Total Usage		
Used Days >= 4 hrs : **40**	Used Days < 4 hrs : **2**	% Used Days >= 4 hrs : **95**
Days not used: **0**	Total days: **42**	Total hours used: **324:16**
Median daily usage: **8:06**	Average daily usage: **7.43**	

Fig. 6.6 The screen of the CPAP statistical report extracted from the equipment and visualized in the ResScan™ system. We observe in these data the patient CPAP statistical report at the 42-day period of CPAP use, after the data presented in Table 6.1. OSA severity is defined as mild for the apnea-hypopnea index (AHI) ≥ 5 and < 15, moderate for AHI ≥ 15 and ≤ 30, and severe for AHI > 30/hr. The patient's mean AHI over this 42-day period of CPAP use was 16.9 events per hour (dotted circle), indicating moderate sleep apnea. (Source: Author's collection)

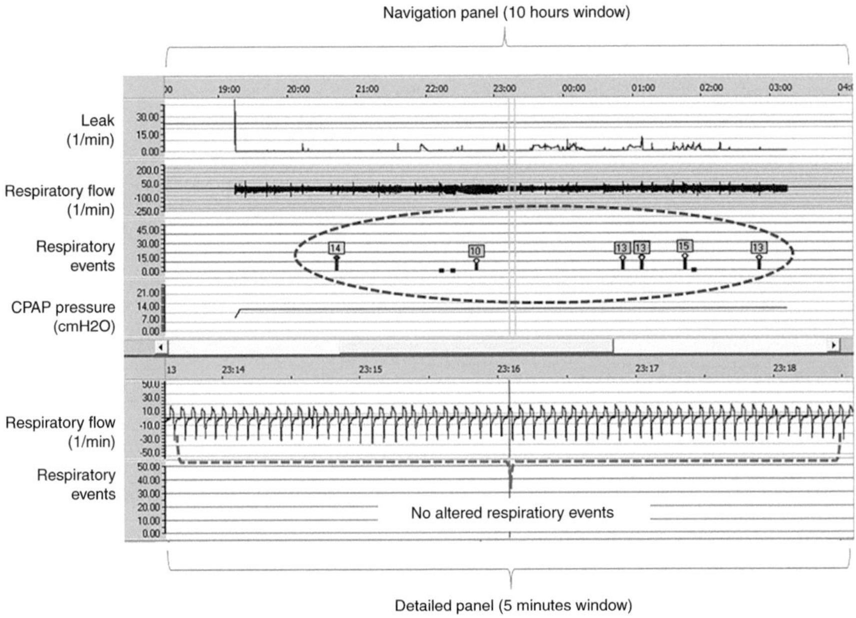

Fig. 6.7 The screen of a graphical data presentation for the ResScan™ system, extracted from positive pressure equipment from ResMed company. We observe few residual respiratory events (dotted circle) and no significant impaired respiratory events in the respiratory flow curve. (Source: Author's collection)

It is important to note that when the patient suffered a stroke, he became more reliant on help, including for positioning during sleep. Checking the patient care schedule, we observed that the nights when he was presenting many residual respiratory events were exactly the nights when a new member of the care team was on duty. This practical nurse placed the patient in a supine position all night long. We emphasize the need for lateral (left or right) supine positioning. After this small positional interference, we observed again the control of residual respiratory events (Table 6.2).

Take Away Message

1. The breathing pattern of a patient with sleep apnea may change over time due to a number of factors. In this case report, it was due to a stroke, but a body weight increase or decrease, chronic obstructive pulmonary diseases among others, could also influence breathing pattern change over the years. A healthcare professional should always be aware of that.
2. Treatment includes identifying the underlying causes.
3. The use of combined therapies can be a simple and cost-effective way to manage sleep apnea. In this case report, positional therapy was associated with PAP therapy to enhance the outcomes of PAP therapy.

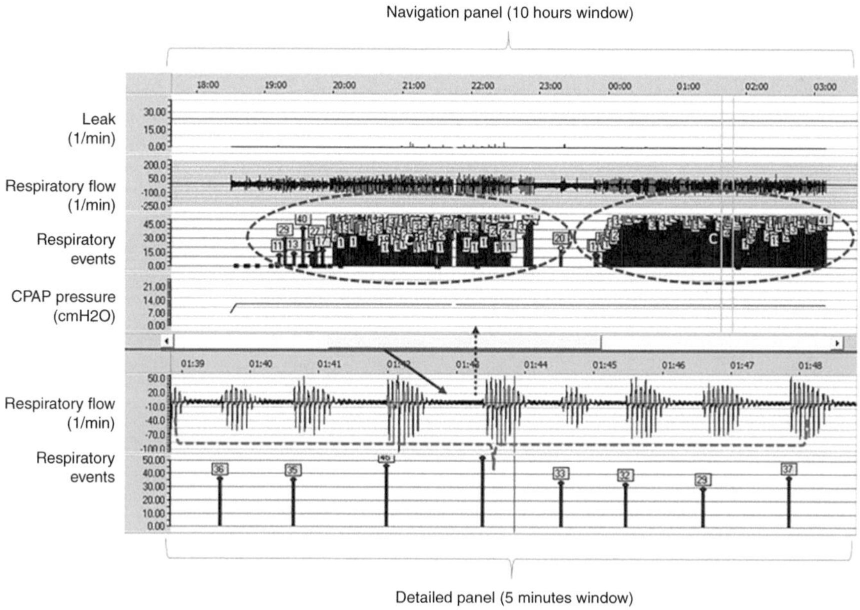

Fig. 6.8 The screen of a graphical data presentation for the ResScan™ system, extracted from positive pressure equipment from ResMed company. In the top window, we can see numerous residual respiratory events (dotted circle), presented by the CPAP algorithm as obstructive respiratory events. At the 5-minute window, we can observe a more detailed respiratory flow curve, signaling characteristics of mixed sleep apnea, such as a progressive decrease (black arrow) and an abrupt increase of the inspiratory curve (dotted arrow) at the end of the apnea event. (Source: Author's collection)

Table 6.2 Presents the main findings of the 47-day period of CPAP use, following appropriate sleep positioning guidelines (right or left side). We can observe a good control of residual AHI (5.2 event/hour). OSA severity is defined as mild for the apnea-hypopnea index (AHI) ≥ 5 and < 15, moderate for AHI ≥ 15 and ≤ 30, and severe for AHI > 30/h. (1) (Source: Author's collection)

	47 days-period of CPAP usage
Days of use/total days (percentile of over 4 h of use per night)	45/47 (91%)
Mask	Oronasal
Pressure—cmH_2O	12.0
Average usage (total number of days)—hours	6:33
Median use (days used)—Hours.	7:11
Expiratory relief	2/only ramp
95th percentile leakage—L/min	0.0
Median leakage—L/min.	4.8
Events per hour (residual AHI)	5.2
Central apnea index	0.6
Obstructive apnea index	0.1
Obstructive hypopnea index	3.9
Unknown apnea index	0.0

References

1. Epstein LJ, Kristo D, Strollo PJ, Friedman N, Malhotra A, Patil SP, et al. Clinical guideline for the evaluation, management and long-term care of obstructive sleep apnea in adults. J Clin Sleep Med. 2009;5(3):263–76.
2. Berry RB, Brooks R, Gamaldo C, Harding SM, Lloyd RM, Quan SF, et al. AASM scoring manual updates for 2017 (version 2.4). J Clin Sleep Med. 2017;13(5):665–6. https://doi.org/10.5664/jcsm.6576.
3. Berry RBBR, Gamaldo CE, Harding SM, Marcus CL, Vaughn BV, Tangredi MM, for the American Academy of Sleep Medicine. The AASM manual for the scoring of sleep and associated events: rules, terminology and technical specifications. Darien, IL: www.aasmnet.org; 2012.

Chapter 7
Case Report: Microarousals Due to Respiratory Effort

7.1 Patient Information

A 69-year-old female, BMI 29.64 kg/m^2, with hypothyroidism, bilateral carotid stents, gastroesophageal reflux, idiopathic pulmonary fibrosis, and mild COPD with moderate restrictive ventilation defect (Fig. 7.1), using oxygen therapy (1 L/min via O_2 cylinder) at night.

At the fourth dose of the COVID-19 vaccine, she had an exacerbation of respiratory symptoms, with dyspnea worsening and coughing. For this reason, patient started a respiratory rehabilitation program (that included two weekly sessions, with PowerBreathe® inspiratory muscle training, aerobic training on a treadmill with oxygen supplementation by nasal cannula at 1260 mL/min of 90% oxygen (INOGEN One G5 portable oxygen concentrator), strength for lower and upper limbs, in addition to functional and flexibility exercises). Six months after initiating the rehabilitation program, there was a significant improvement in respiratory symptoms. Despite the improvement, the patient complained of fatigue and daytime sleepiness and was submitted to polysomnography.

Diagnostic polysomnography (Fig. 7.2) showed a marked increase in the apnea/hypopnea index (87.4/h) with central apneas (8.3/h), mixed apneas (13.8/h), obstructive apneas (17.6/h), and a predominance of hypopneas (47.7/h), with a maximum duration of 29.5 s. Also was observed periods of cyclical change in respiratory amplitude, in an increasing/decreasing range suggestive of Cheyne-Stokes respiration (however, it is important to point out that, depending on the position, central apneas may arise due to obstruction of the upper airways because of the posterior displacement of the tongue base by gravity action) [1]. Basal saturation was 92%, and severe desaturation of oxyhemoglobin associated with breathing events was observed. Sometimes there was no saturation improvement during the inter-apnea

V. S. Piccin, *Monitoring Positive Pressure Therapy in Sleep-Related Breathing Disorders*, https://doi.org/10.1007/978-3-031-50292-7_7

		Ref	LLN	Pre Meas	Pre % Ref	Post Meas	Post % Ref	Post % Chg
VC	Liters	2.82	2.18	1.63	58	1.55	55	-5
FVC	Liters	2.82	2.18	1.44	51	1.34	48	-6
FEV1	Liters	2.21	1.60	1.19	54	1.13	51	-5
FEV1/FVC	%	78	70	83	106	84	107	1
FEV1/SVC	%			73		73		-0
FEF25-75%	L/sec	2.04	1.16	1.77	87	1.65	81	-7
FET25-75%	Sec	0.80	0.47	0.41	51	0.41	51	0
PEF	L/sec	6.74	5.05	5.03	75	6.14	91	22
FEF75%	L/sec	0.67	0.36	0.38	56	0.40	59	5
FEF/FIF50		<1.00		1.51		1.52		1

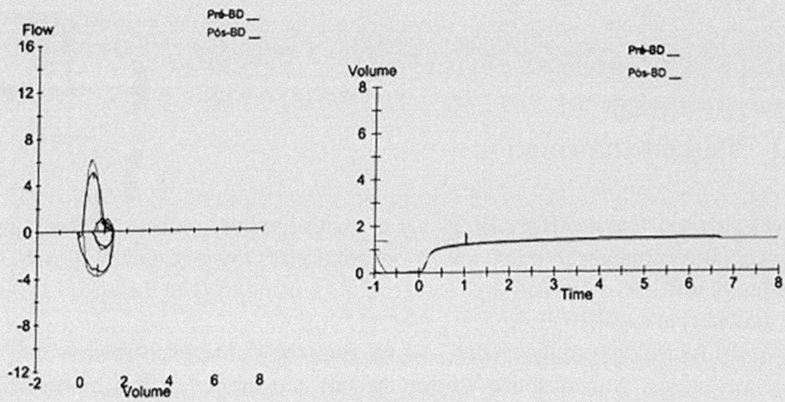

Fig. 7.1 Spirometry examination with moderate restrictive ventilation defect (no response to bronchodilator). *FVC* forced vital capacity, *FEV1* forced expiratory volume in 1 s, *FEF* forced expiratory flow, *PEF* peak expiratory flow, *SVC* slow vital capacity, *FET* forced expiratory time, *FIF* forced inspiratory flow, *LLN* lower limit of normal

period. The mean saturation during the night was 86%, and at 29% of the total sleep time the saturation level remained below 85%, reaching a minimal saturation of 63%. The patient exhibited intense and consistent snoring, important sleep fragmentation, normal latency for sleep onset (13.5 min), and reduced REM sleep latency (37.0 min). Sleep effectiveness was normal (94.4%). Sleep architecture presented a reduction in REM sleep (N1–3.0%; N2–53.9%; N3–24.7%; REM—18.4%). PSG was carried out in ambient air to enhance the evaluation of respiratory events. The study was consistent with severe sleep apnea with periods of Cheyne-Stokes breathing. Epworth Sleepiness Scale: 14.

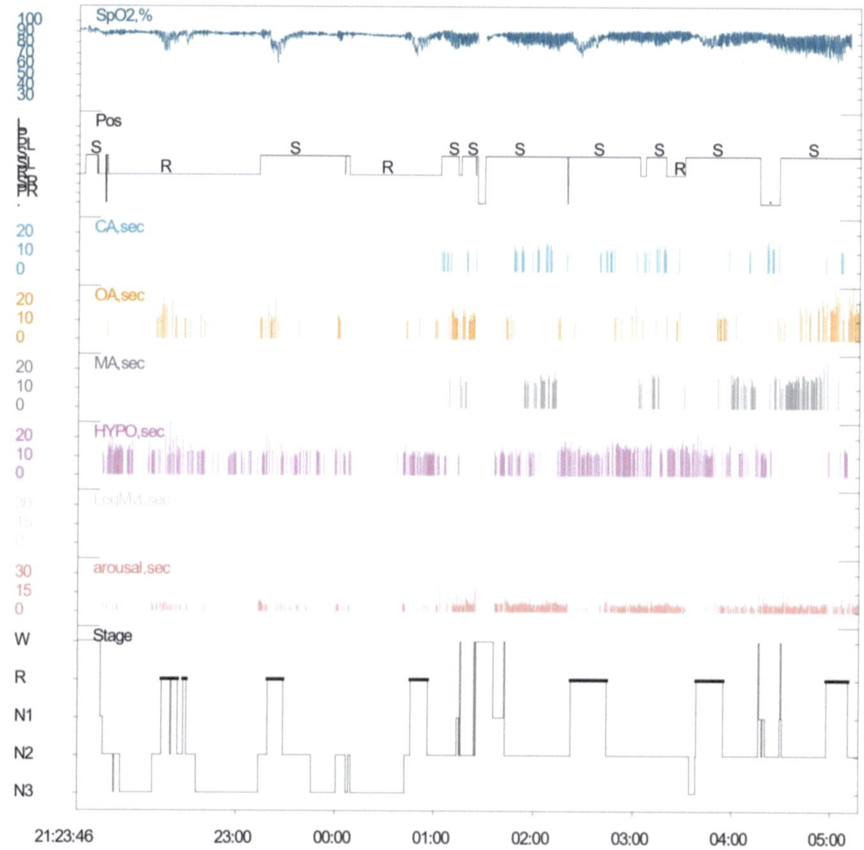

Fig. 7.2 Patient hypnogram derived from polysomnographic examination showing SaO2: Oxygen Saturation; Stage: Sleep Stage; W: Vigil; REM: REM sleep; N1: stage 1; N2: Stage 2; N3: Stage 3; *CA* Central Apnea, *Sec* duration in seconds, *OA* obstructive apnea, *MA* mixed apnea, *Hypo* Hypopnea, *Arousal* awakening, *LegMVT* leg movement, *Pos* body position, *R* right lateral decubitus, *S* supine, *P* prone

7.2 Therapeutic Intervention

The patient started PAP therapy by using fixed CPAP (9.0 cmH_2O) plus oxygen therapy (1 L/min via O_2 cylinder) with nasal mask (YN-02 YUWELL Nasal Vented Mask with forehead support). Upon medical advice, the patient has been using bed head elevation (approximately 12 cm) for 3 years prior to starting CPAP.

In a three-month evaluation of CPAP use, the patient presented a residual IAH of 0.4 events/hour, 8:10 h of average daily CPAP usage, percentile 95 leakage was 25.2 L/min (median leakage of 0.0 L/min), and 98% of CPAP usage more than 4 h in that period. On the other hand, the patient began to exhibit hypertensive peaks of undefined cause.

The 24-h Ambulatory Blood Pressure Monitoring (ABPM) test revealed hypertension during sleep (Table 7.1).

In the analysis of the respiratory flow curve (Fig. 7.3), numerous periods of flattening of the inspiratory flow curve were observed, using a fixed CPAP of 9.0 cmH_2O. This suggests that hypertension could be attributed to suboptimal CPAP

Table 7.1 Presents the 24-Hour Ambulatory Blood Pressure Monitoring (ABPM), before and after corticoid intake reduction (where there was a significant blood pressure improvement). Thresholds for having high blood pressure (BP) on ABPM were defined as follows: ≥130/80 mm Hg for daytime BP, ≥ 125/75 mm Hg for 24-hour BP, and ≥ 110/65 mm Hg for nighttime BP [2]. SBP: Systolic blood pressure; DBP: Diastolic blood pressure. Source: Author's collection

	1st ABPM	2nd ABPM (after corticoid intake reduction)
Systolic blood pressure		
24 h	143 mmHg	122 mmHg
Daytime	138 mmHg	120 mmHg
Night-time	159 mmHg	129 mmHg
Night-time fall in SBP (%)	15%	7%
Diastolic blood pressure		
24 h	93 mmHg	80 mmHg
Daytime	91 mmHg	78 mmHg
Night-time	99 mmHg	89 mmHg
Night-time fall in DBP (%)	9%	13%

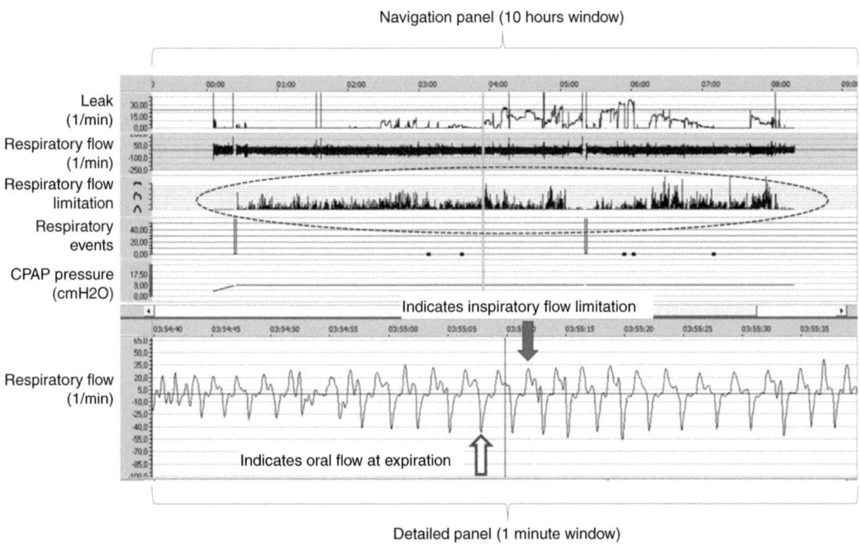

Fig. 7.3 Screen of a graphical data presentation for the ResScan™ system, extracted from positive pressure equipment by ResMed company, at fixed pressure of 9.0 cmH_2O. In the upper window, we can see numerous respiratory flow limitation events (dotted circle). In the 5-min window, we can observe a more detailed respiratory flow curve, indicating limitation of the inspiratory flow curve (gray arrow) and exhalation tracing suggestive of airflow leakage through the mouth (white arrow). (Source: author's collection)

(causing increased respiratory effort, microarousals, and activation of the sympathetic nervous system) [3]. The CPAP was adjusted to 9.4 cmH_2O, but with no hypertension improvement and no flattening resolution of the inspiratory flow curve.

In addition, the search for other possible causes of the patient's increased blood pressure has begun. We identified that the patient was using Prednisone (60 mg/day) for the treatment of a previous flu condition. The patient was already using low doses of corticosteroids for pulmonary fibrosis. She had the flu and was medicated with an increased dose of corticosteroids for a short period of time. Inadvertently, she continued to use the high dose even after the influenza had resolved. The literature shows an inter-relationship between taking corticosteroids and high blood pressure. The underlying pathophysiological mechanisms are not well understood [4, 5]. The mechanisms of corticoid-induced hypertension include increased systemic vascular resistance, increased extracellular volume, and increased cardiac contractility [6]. So the doctor started to wean off the corticoid intake.

In the same period, new adjustments were made to the CPAP pressure (fixed pressure at 9.8 cmH_2O) for gradual correction of respiratory flow restrictions during sleep. The patient did not present any specific complaint regarding pressure therapy during these adjustments and therapeutic results were excellent (Table 7.2), but still inspiratory flow limitation was observed at respiratory flow curve analysis (Fig. 7.4).

Table 7.2 Presents the main results of CPAP use at fixed pressure of 9.0, 9.4, 9.8, and 10.0 cmH_2O respectively. A good control of the residual AHI can be observed in each fitted pressure. Furthermore, no patient complains at these different levels of CPAP pressure (although the leak was greater when using the nasal mask without forehead support). OSA severity is defined as mild for apnea-hypopnea index (AHI) ≥ 5 and < 15, moderate for AHI ≥ 15 and ≤ 30, and severe for AHI > 30/h [7, 8]. Source: Author's collection

Variables	CPAP use at 9.0 cmH_2O	CPAP use at 9.4 cmH_2O	CPAP use at 9.8 cmH_2O	CPAP use at 10.0 cmH_2O
Usage days/total days (percentile of more than 4 h of usage per night)	205/1 (97%)	11/0 (100%)	70/5 (91%)	9/0 (100%)
Mask	Nasal with forehead	Nasal with forehead	Nasal with forehead	Nasal without forehead
Average usage (total days) – Hours	7:55	8:05	7:22	9:04
Median usage (days used) - hours	7:59	7:51	7:45	8:41
Expiratory relief	Off	Off	Off	Off
95th percentile leaks – L/min	25.2	15.6	22.8	31.2
Median leaks – L/min	0.0	0.0	0.0	0.0
Events per hour (residual AHI)	0.5	0.6	0.5	0.6
Central apnea index	0.0	0.0	0.0	0.0
Obstructive apnea index	0.0	0.0	0.0	0.0
Obstructive hypopnea index	0.2	0.2	0.2	0.2
Unknown apnea index	0.2	0.3	0.2	0.2

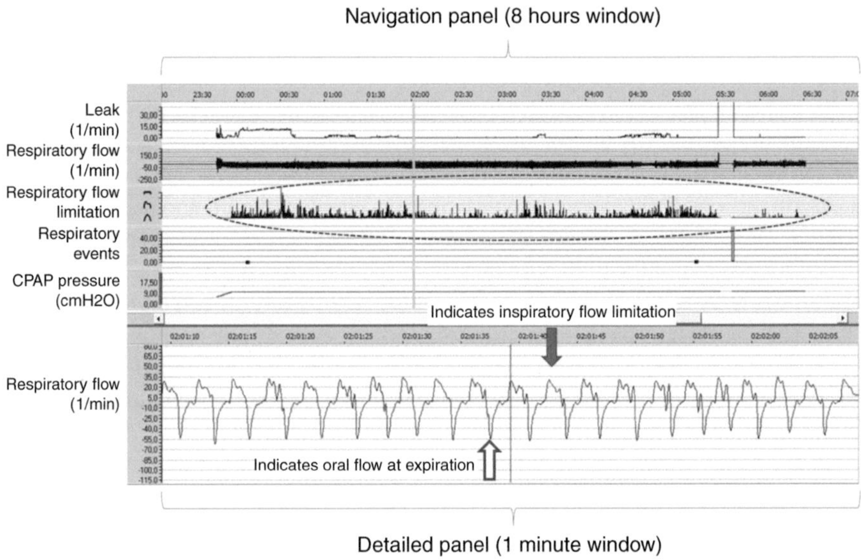

Fig. 7.4 Screen of a graphical data presentation for the ResScan™ system, extracted from positive pressure equipment by ResMed company, at fixed pressure of 9.8 cmH_2O. In the upper window, comparing with Fig. 7.3, we can observe less events of respiratory flow limitation (dotted circle). In the 5-min window, also comparing with Fig. 7.3, we can observe the detailed respiratory flow curve, indicating less limitation of the inspiratory flow curve (gray arrow) and exhalation tracing suggestive of less airflow leakage through the mouth (white arrow). (Source: author's collection)

Unfortunately, after 2 weeks of reduced corticosteroid intake, the patient suffered an exacerbation of respiratory symptoms, initiating antibiotic therapy at home. Less than a month after the onset of respiratory symptoms, she was hospitalized for pseudo-membranous colitis, lung congestion, and hypervolemia treatment.

The patient stayed at the hospital for about 10 days. After hospital discharge, the patient returned to the pulmonary rehabilitation program, dependent on full-time additional O_2 supply (oxygen supplementation by nasal cannula at 420–630 mL/min of 90% oxygen (INOGEN One G5 portable oxygen concentrator)). She underwent the ABPM exam again, which showed improvement in blood pressure levels compared to the previous exam (Table 7.1).

In a short time, the patient was weaned from the use of additional daytime oxygen. As the respiratory flow curve restriction events continued during sleep, a new pressure setting was performed on the CPAP equipment (fixed pressure at 10.0 cmH_2O). With the pressure increase we observed much less events of respiratory flow limitation, a better amplitude of the respiratory flow curve, and almost no signal of air leak through the mouth (Fig. 7.5).

For additional information, the nasal mask was replaced, due to usage damage, with the YN-03 YUWELL Nasal Vented mask (without forehead support, as shown in Fig. 7.6).

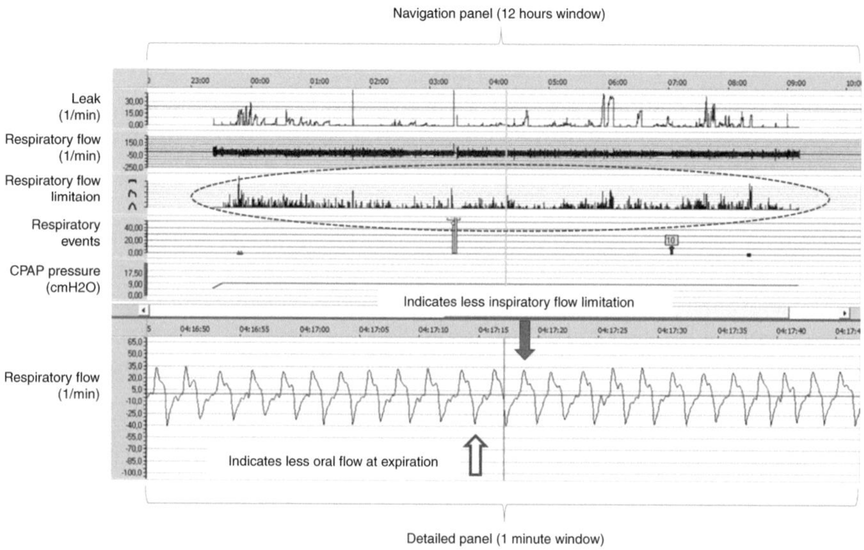

Fig. 7.5 Screen of a graphical data presentation for the ResScan™ system, extracted from positive pressure equipment by ResMed company, at fixed pressure of 10.0 cmH_2O. In the upper window, although we can observe respiratory flow limitation events (dotted circle), these events are less present in relation to Figs. 7.3 and 7.4. In the 5-min window, we can observe a better amplitude of the respiratory flow curve, indicating less limitation of the inspiratory flow curve (gray arrow) and expiratory tracing suggestive of resolution of the air leak through the mouth (white arrow). (Source: author's collection)

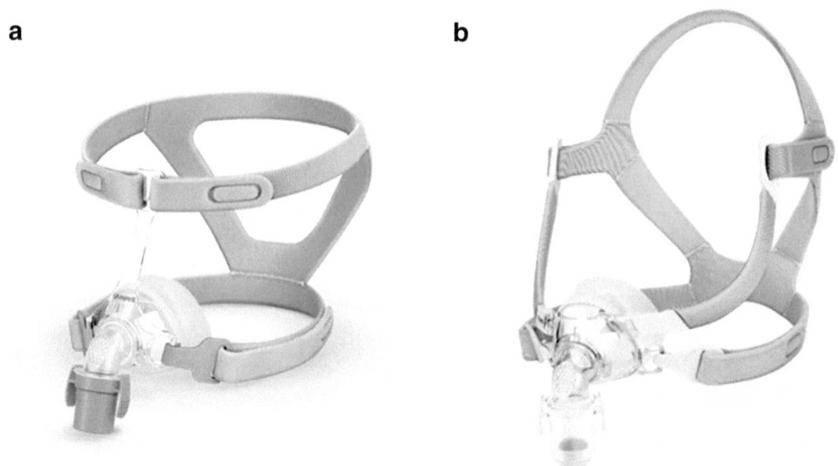

Fig. 7.6 (**a**) Nasal mask YN-02 from Yuwell; (**b**) Nasal mask YN-03 from Yuwell. It can be observed that the main difference between these two models of nasal masks is the front support. Source: author collection

No difference was found in the main results of using CPAP at a fixed pressure of 9.0, 9.4, 9.8, and 10.0 cmH_2O respectively (Table 7.2). Interestingly, both the first and second ABPM were performed with the same CPAP pressure level (fixed pressure at 9.8 cmH_2O), but the second ABPM showed a reduction in blood pressure even with the restriction of the respiratory flow curve observed in Fig. 7.4 (which is a representative graphic example of the flow curve with CPAP pressure fixed at 9.8 cmH_2O).

There is increasing evidence that mean nocturnal blood pressure (BP) is an important indicator of cardiovascular morbidity and mortality [9]. Any disturbance in the sleep quality is a mechanism through which a sympathetic tone increases in and, in turn, an increase in BP may occur. The way auto-CPAP works can induce micro-arousals from inappropriate increases in pressure due to changing positions, after a central apnea, during a period of flow limitation or, more often, without any identifiable reason [10]. Studies have shown a greater impact of fixed-CPAP on 24 h diastolic blood pressure compared with auto-CPAP [10]. Researchers also demonstrated that auto-CPAP devices did not improve heart rate variability, while fixed-CPAP did [10]. These statements justify our strategy of using fixed-CPAP in this clinical case.

As we observed, there is still room for improvement with regard to the patient's blood pressure during the night, even with the reduction in blood pressure obtained with the removal of corticosteroid. The flattening of the inspiratory flow is related to resistance of the airway, which can occur even with application of positive airway pressure, and may be the causal factor of the lack of blood pressure control [11]. On the other hand, respiratory flow limitation is often not detected/displayed in the statistical report of positive pressure equipment. Titration of CPAP through analysis of the respiratory flow curve to eliminate flow limitation may be associated with improved clinical outcomes, compared to the treatment of apneas and hypopneas only.

Take Away Message

1. A limitation of respiratory flow during sleep can be present even if the equipment's statistical report indicates the resolution of respiratory events.
2. Respiratory flow limitation can increase microarousals due to respiratory effort, resulting in activation of the sympathetic nervous system during sleep and impairing the fall in blood pressure during the night.
3. However, it is not necessarily the sole causal factor that influences the pressure drop during sleep. The potential hypertensive action of medications should also be studied.
4. Advanced graphic data evaluation, and especially the respiratory flow curve evaluation for CPAP patients, is a conduct that should be introduced in the follow-up of patients, especially for the most challenging cases. The interpretation of the flow curve may provide important data for therapeutic appropriateness and management.

References

1. Issa FG, Sullivan CE. Reversal of central sleep apnea using nasal CPAP. Chest. 1986;90(2):165–71. https://doi.org/10.1378/chest.90.2.165.
2. Muntner P, Carey RM, Jamerson K, Wright JT, Whelton PK. Rationale for ambulatory and home blood pressure monitoring thresholds in the 2017 American College of Cardiology/ American Heart Association guideline. Hypertension. 2019;73(1):33–8. https://doi.org/10.1161/HYPERTENSIONAHA.118.11946.
3. Calero G, Farre R, Ballester E, Hernandez L, Daniel N, Montserrat Canal JM. Physiological consequences of prolonged periods of flow limitation in patients with sleep apnea hypopnea syndrome. Respir Med. 2006;100(5):813–7. https://doi.org/10.1016/j.rmed.2005.09.016.
4. Rice JB, White AG, Scarpati LM, Wan G, Nelson WW. Long-term systemic corticosteroid exposure: a systematic literature review. Clin Ther. 2017;39(11):2216–29. https://doi.org/10.1016/j.clinthera.2017.09.011.
5. Fardet L, Flahault A, Kettaneh A, Tiev KP, Généreau T, Tolédano C, et al. Corticosteroid-induced clinical adverse events: frequency, risk factors and patient's opinion. Br J Dermatol. 2007;157(1):142–8. https://doi.org/10.1111/j.1365-2133.2007.07950.x.
6. Schäcke H, Döcke WD, Asadullah K. Mechanisms involved in the side effects of glucocorticoids. Pharmacol Ther. 2002;96(1):23–43. https://doi.org/10.1016/s0163-7258(02)00297-8.
7. Berry RB, Brooks R, Gamaldo C, Harding SM, Lloyd RM, Quan SF, et al. AASM scoring manual updates for 2017 (version 2.4). J Clin Sleep Med. 2017;13(5):665–6. https://doi.org/10.5664/jcsm.6576.
8. Berry RBBR, Gamaldo CE, Harding SM, Marcus CL, Vaughn BV, Tangredi MM, for the American Academy of Sleep Medicine. The AASM manual for the scoring of sleep and associated events: rules, terminology and technical specifications. Darien, IL: www.aasmnet.org; 2012.
9. Thunström E, Manhem K, Rosengren A, Peker Y. Blood pressure response to losartan and continuous positive airway pressure in hypertension and obstructive sleep apnea. Am J Respir Crit Care Med. 2016;193(3):310–20. https://doi.org/10.1164/rccm.201505-0998OC.
10. Pépin JL, Tamisier R, Baguet JP, Lepaulle B, Arbib F, Arnol N, et al. Fixed-pressure CPAP versus auto-adjusting CPAP: comparison of efficacy on blood pressure in obstructive sleep apnoea, a randomised clinical trial. Thorax. 2016;71(8):726–33. https://doi.org/10.1136/thoraxjnl-2015-207700.
11. Arora N, Meskill G, Guilleminault C. The role of flow limitation as an important diagnostic tool and clinical finding in mild sleep-disordered breathing. Sleep Sci. 2015;8(3):134–42. https://doi.org/10.1016/j.slsci.2015.08.003.

Chapter 8
Case Report: Positional Sleep Apnea

8.1 Patient Information

An 82-year-old male, BMI 31.2 kg/m^2, modified Mallampati scale: 4, SaO_2 93% and HR 58 bpm, at rest. A history of knee replacement surgery, four cardiac stents, removal of a prostate tumor, phimosis surgery, and mandibular splint. In addition, he has been diagnosed with mild Parkinson's disease, with impaired mobility, restricted walking, and is dependent for activities of daily living. The patient uses levothyroxine, levodopa, fluvoxamine, rasagiline, indapamide, amiodarone, cilostazol, acetylsalicylic acid, allopurinol, atenolol, rosuvastatine calcium, quetiapine, chondroitin, mineral antioxidant supplement and vitamin D. Low alcohol intake (wine, once a week) and moderate daily physical activity (twice a week, with physical therapist). Ex-smoker (stopped smoking 35 years ago, before the patient was exposed to 50 packets-years of smoke).

The patient reports that he usually goes to bed at 10 PM. and wakes up at 6 AM. Due to daytime drowsiness problems (Epworth scale: 11) and sudden elevated blood pressure, the patient underwent diagnostic polysomnography. The exam started at 10:16:33 pm and ended at 07:32:03 am. The patient presented a sleep latency of 6.5 min and elevated REM latency (265.5 min). The total sleep time (TST) was 363.0 min, with a sleep efficiency of 65.3%. The sleep stage distribution was 20.7% stage N1, 59.2% stage N2, 0.0% stage N3, and 20.1% REM sleep. The waking time after falling asleep was 176.5 min. There were 297 awakenings, an average of 49.1 per hour. The index of periodic limb movements during sleep was 0.0 per hour. In total, 524 respiratory events were reported, including 283 obstructive apneas, 28 central apneas, 89 mixed apneas, and 124 obstructive hypopneas. The respiratory disturbance index (RDI) was 86.6 per hour, and the apnea/hypopnea index (AHI) was 86.6 per hour. Basal oxyhemoglobin saturation was 92%, mean SaO_2 of 89%, and minimum SaO_2 of 63%. The desaturation index was 74.8 per hour

V. S. Piccin, *Monitoring Positive Pressure Therapy in Sleep-Related Breathing Disorders*, https://doi.org/10.1007/978-3-031-50292-7_8

during REM sleep and 63.5 per hour during NREM sleep. SaO_2 has remained below 90% for 51.7% of total registration time. The patient hypnogram is shown in Fig. 8.1.

Following the findings of the polysomnographic exam, the patient was referred for PAP treatment. Initiated PAP therapy using auto CPAP (5.4–10.0 cmH_2O) with an oronasal mask Quattro Fx ResMed large (patient was unable to adapt to a nasal mask due to excessive oral leakage and discomfort). Table 8.1 shows the results of the first week of CPAP use.

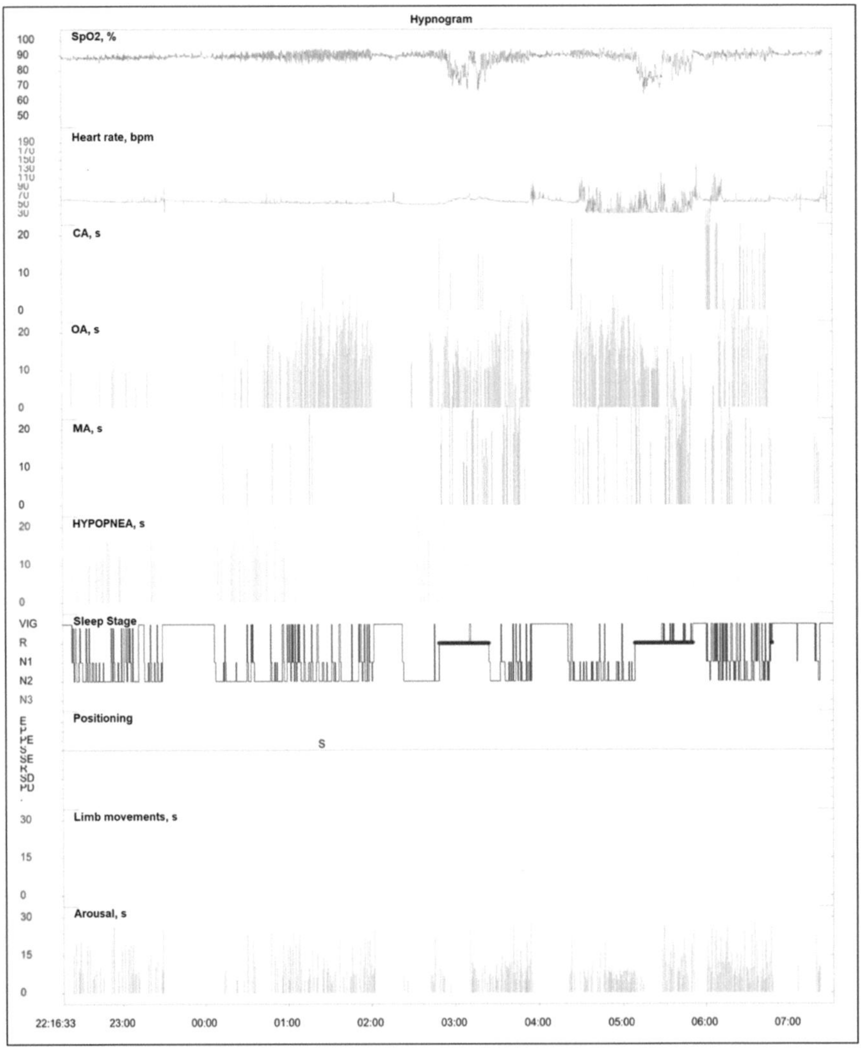

Fig. 8.1 Hypnogram of the patient from a polysomnographic exam showing sleep fragmentation, desaturation, and hypopnea events throughout the night

Table 8.1 Presents the main results of the 7-day period of CPAP usage. We can observe a lack of control of the residual AHI (36.8 event/h). OSA severity is defined as mild for apnea-hypopnea index (AHI) ≥ 5 and < 15, moderate for AHI ≥ 15 and ≤ 30, and severe for AHI > 30/h [1, 2]. Source: Author's collection

	7 days-period of CPAP usage
Usage days/total days (percentile of more than 4 h of usage per night)	7/7 (100%)
Mask	Oronasal
Pressure—cmH_2O	5.4–10.0
Average usage (total days)—Hours	9:53
Median usage (days used)—hours	9:26
Expiratory relief	Off
95th percentile leaks—L/min	15.6
Median leaks—L/min	3.6
Events per hour (residual AHI)	**36.8**
Central apnea index	0.7
Obstructive apnea index	**34.5**
Obstructive hypopnea index	1.6
Unknown apnea index	0.0

8.2 Therapeutic Intervention

In the first week of CPAP use, the patient showed good adherence parameters (the American Association of Sleep Medicine—AASM considers adequate adherence to use CPAP for more than 4 hours per night on at least 70% of nights during the period evaluated) [3]. However, positive pressure therapy was not effective in normalizing the patient's AHI. In the analysis of the respiratory flow curve, concentrated periods of periodic respiration were observed, which lasted only the first half of the night (Fig. 8.2). After investigation with the patient's family, it was possible to verify that the patient was commonly positioned in the supine position in the first half of the night and, in the second half, placed in the lateral decubitus to prevent positioning bedsores.

The change in bed position explained the difference in the breathing pattern observed in the second half of the night (Fig. 8.3), and is in line with what had already been verified in previous studies that demonstrated that the threshold to upper airway collapse by negative inspiratory pressure is decreased in the supine posture compared with the lateral position in patients with OSA [4].

The patient's family was asked to proceed with positioning therapy without placing the patient in a supine position. In addition, the CPAP pressure range was also increased by the previous observation of certain limitation periods in the inspiratory flow curve, even with the patient in lateral decubitus. After these procedures, therapeutic success was observed (Table 8.2), with good control of respiratory events during sleep, comfort for the patient, and reduction of his cognitive and motor limitations.

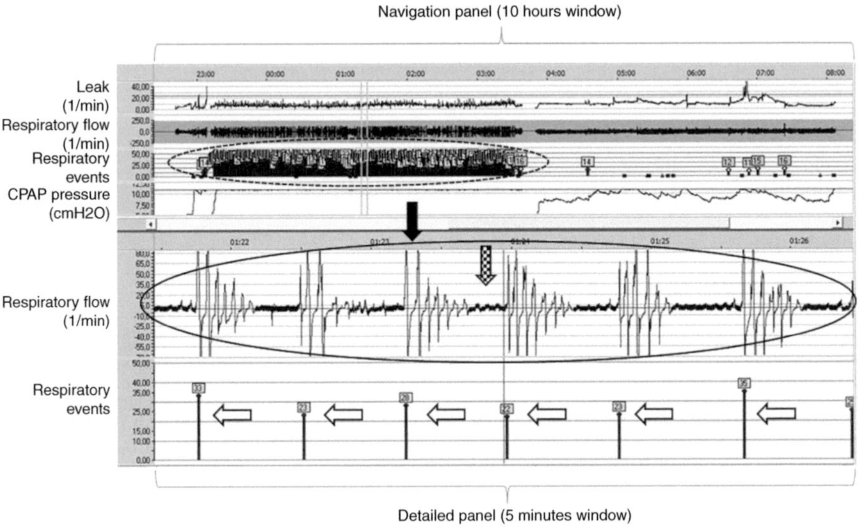

Fig. 8.2 In the analysis of the respiratory flow curve, concentrated periods of periodic breathing were observed, lasting only in the first half of the night (dashed circle). The CPAP algorithm identifies the events as obstructive apnea events (open arrow). But, when observing the beginning of the respiratory event, there are periods of hyperventilation (closed arrow) followed for apneas (checked arrow) and ending with another hyperventilation event (usually, this flow curve pattern indicates that a mixed apnea occurred. Source: author collection

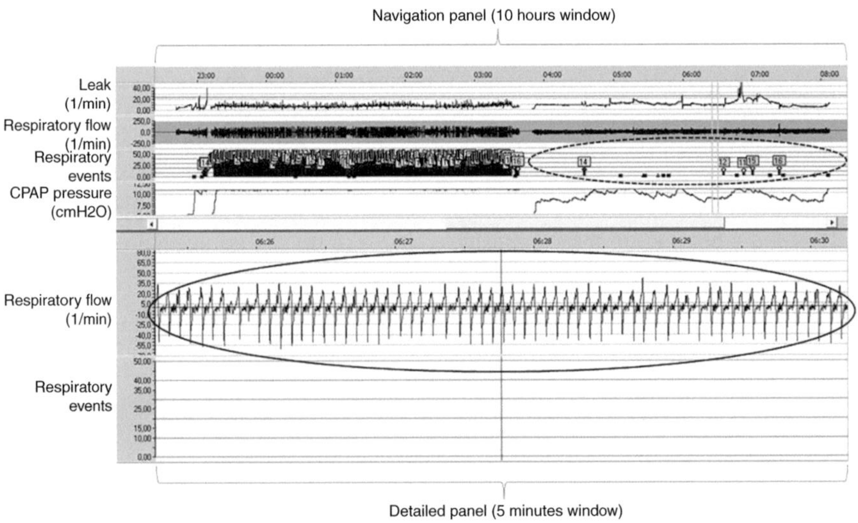

Fig. 8.3 In the analysis of the respiratory flow curve the second half of the night, there are no concentrated periods of periodic breathing (dashed circle). The CPAP algorithm found no obstructive apnea events as in Fig. 8.2 (closed circle). (Source: author collection)

Table 8.2 Presents the main results of the 18 days-period of CPAP usage. We can observe a good control of residual AHI (4.3 event/h). OSA severity is defined as mild for apnea-hypopnea index (AHI) ≥ 5 and < 15, moderate for AHI ≥ 15 and ≤ 30, and severe for AHI > 30/h [1, 2]. Source: Author's collection

	18 days-period of CPAP usage
Usage days/total days (percentile of more than 4 hours of usage per night)	18/18 (88%)
Mask	Oronasal
Pressure—cmH_2O	5.6–13.0
Average usage (total days)—Hours	6:43
Median usage (days used)—hours	7:32
Expiratory relief	Off
95th percentile leaks—L/min	25.8
Median leaks—L/min	1.8
Events per hour (residual AHI)	4.3
Central apnea index	0.4
Obstructive apnea index	1.3
Obstructive hypopnea index	2.1
Unknown apnea index	0.0

After initiating pressure therapy, the patient reported that he began walking longer distances and with less fatigue. The patient reported an improvement in his mood and vitality, restorative sleep, and improvement in daytime fatigue. He also indicated that he could perform daily activities that he previously had trouble with. Her family also mentioned that the patient had improved physically.

Take Away Message

1. Anatomical factors combined with body position during sleep can alter respiratory patterns throughout the night. In this case, the supine position was the causal factor in the residual obstructive events during sleep, probably due to the action of gravity on the base of the tongue and soft palate.
2. It is important to note that certain patients tend to sleep more in the supine position during PSG than during home sleep, so a one-night sleep study may be insufficient and may overestimate the severity of OSA in these individuals. As the patient in this case remained only supine in the PSG, this may have overestimated the severity of his sleep apnea.
3. Increasing CPAP pressure is not always the way to improve supine breathing (as increased pressure can cause discomfort, central respiratory events, and increased leakage).
4. Identifying external factors that may affect the patient's breathing is of fundamental importance for the proper conduct of the airway pressure adaptation program.
5. Evaluation of high-resolution graphical data and sleep flow curves is a low-cost and highly beneficial procedure for the proper performance of positive airway pressure therapy.

References

1. Berry RBBR, Gamaldo CE, Harding SM, Marcus CL, Vaughn BV, Tangredi MM, for the American Academy of Sleep Medicine. The AASM manual for the scoring of sleep and associated events: rules, terminology and technical specifications. Darien, IL: www.aasmnet.org; 2012.
2. Berry RB, Brooks R, Gamaldo C, Harding SM, Lloyd RM, Quan SF, et al. AASM scoring manual updates for 2017 (version 2.4). J Clin Sleep Med. 2017;13(5):665–6. https://doi.org/10.5664/jcsm.6576.
3. Kribbs NB, Pack AI, Kline LR, Smith PL, Schwartz AR, Schubert NM, et al. Objective measurement of patterns of nasal CPAP use by patients with obstructive sleep apnea. Am Rev Respir Dis. 1993;147(4):887–95. https://doi.org/10.1164/ajrccm/147.4.887.
4. Issa FG, Sullivan CE. Reversal of central sleep apnea using nasal CPAP. Chest. 1986;90(2):165–71. https://doi.org/10.1378/chest.90.2.165.

Chapter 9
Case Report: Leaking Through the Mouth

9.1 Patient Information

A 64-year-old male, BMI 27.3 kg/m^2, modified Mallampati scale: 4, 95% SaO_2 and HR 65 bpm, at rest. A history of tonsillectomy surgery, non-smoking, drinking-free, and practicing daily physical activity. The patient uses pitavastatine, metformin hydrochloride, latanoprost, and an herbal sleeping pill. The patient reports that he usually goes to bed at 11 PM. and wakes up at 5 AM. For further information, the patient has reported using a mandibular advancement device (MAD) for 10 years.

A previous diagnostic polysomnography was performed using MAD (Fig. 9.1). Examination was carried out in a Nihon Kohden device, with simultaneous electroencephalogram evaluation (F3-M2, C3-M2, O1-M2, F4-M1, C4-M1, O2-M1), electrooculogram, electromyogram (submental region and tibialis anterior muscle), body position, snoring, nasal pressure transducer, effort thoracic and abdominal breathing, arterial oxygen saturation (SaO_2) and electrocardiogram. The total registration time was 428.5 min. Stage N1 latency was 8.5 min (normal <30 min) while REM latency was 115.0 min (normal = 70–120 min). Total sleep time was 364.5 min (85.06% efficiency; normal >85%) and the percentages of sleep phases in relation to the total time of sleep were: N1: 17.7%; N2: 43.1%; N3: 22.1%; REM sleep: 17.1%. Wake-up time after starting sleep was 50 min. There were 175 micro-arousals (duration <15 s), with an index of 28.8/h (normal <10/h). 207 respiratory pauses were recorded during sleep, divided into 79 apneas (79 obstructive, 0 mixed, 0 central), and 128 hypopneas. Basal SaO_2 was 94%, average SaO_2 was 94% and minimum SaO_2 was 80%, with 2.7% of sleep time below 90% of SaO_2. The apnea-hypopnea index (AHI) was 34.1/h (normal <5/h). Heart rate ranged between 49 and 75 bpm (mean 54 bpm), sinus rhythm. No periodical movement of limbs during sleep was observed.

V. S. Piccin, *Monitoring Positive Pressure Therapy in Sleep-Related Breathing Disorders*, https://doi.org/10.1007/978-3-031-50292-7_9

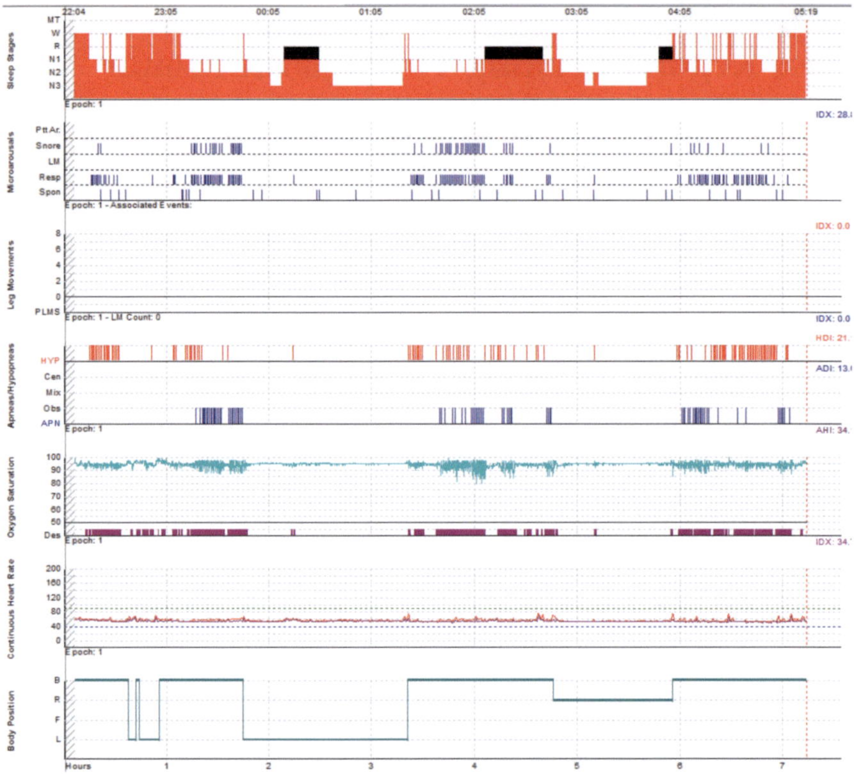

Fig. 9.1 Patient hypnogram derived from polysomnographic examination by using a mandibular advancement device, showing that respiratory events are predominant, albeit not exclusively present in NREMS and at the supine position during sleep. Body position – *R* right lateral decubitus, *B* supine (Back), *F* prone (Front), and *L* left lateral decubitus. (Source: author's collection)

Then a new polysomnography examination without MAD was carried out (Fig. 9.2). The examination was recorded in the Alice 6 LDxS system. Sleep latency was 5.5 min and latency to initiate REM sleep was 80.0 min. Total sleep time (TTS) was 388.5 min, with a sleep efficiency of 87.7%. The sleep stage distribution was 7.7% stage N1, 56.5% stage N2, 19.9% stage N3, and 15.8% REM sleep. Wake-up time after falling asleep was 48.8 min. There were 150 awakenings, with an index of 22.2 (n°/h). The index for the periodical movement of the lower limbs was 0.0 (n°/h), with 0.0 (n°/h) associated with the awakenings. The total number of respiratory events was 172, of which 79 were obstructive apneas, 9 central apneas, 0 mixed apneas, 84 obstructive hypopneas, 0 central hypopneas, and 0 "RERAs". The respiratory disturbance index (RDI) was 26.6 (n°/h) and the apnea/hypopnea index (AHI) 26.6 (no./h). The obstructive apnea/hypopnea index (AHI) was 25.20 (n°/h) and the central apnea/hypopnea (AHC) was 1.40 (n°/h). Basal oxyhemoglobin saturation was 95%, average 92%, and minimum SaO_2 was 76%. The desaturation index was 45.9 (n°/h) during REM sleep and 23.5 (n°/h) during NREM sleep. At 7.7% of the total registration time, SpO_2 stayed below 90%.

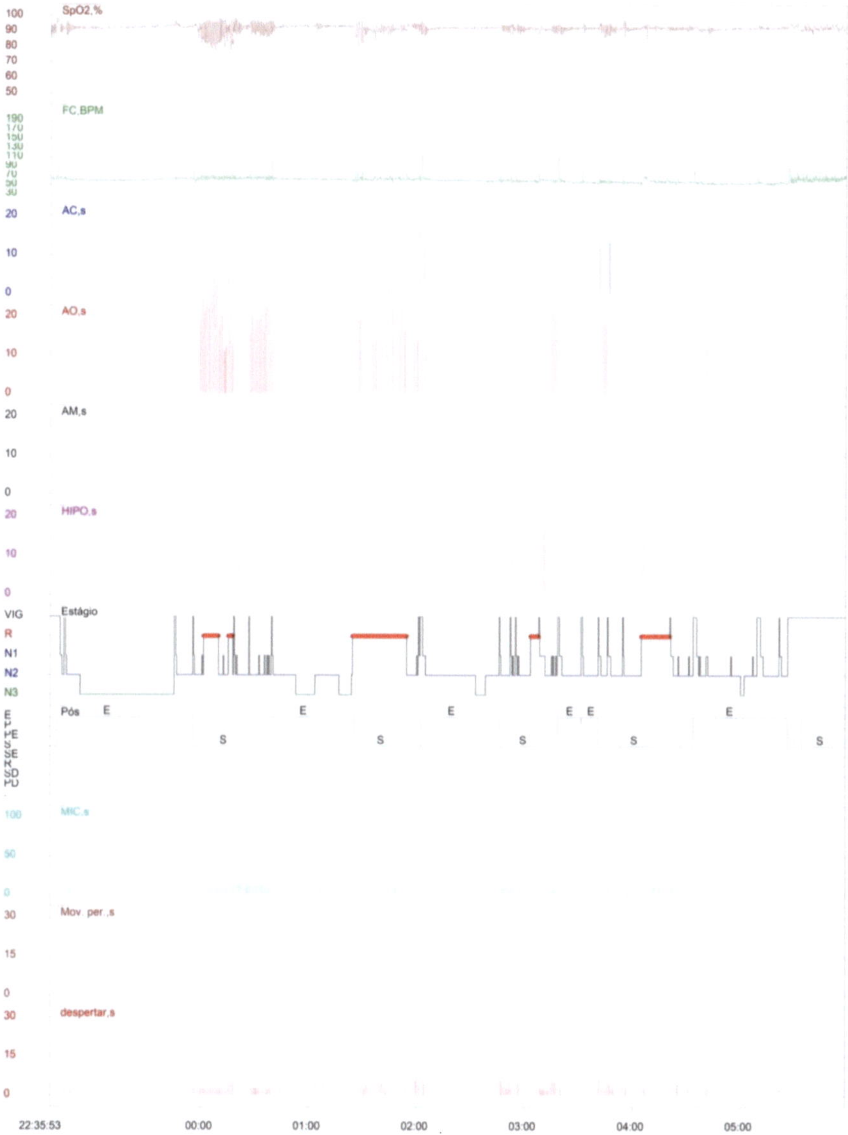

Fig. 9.2 Patient hypnogram derived from a polysomnography exam without a mandibular advancement device. Contrary to Fig. 9.1 respiratory events are not predominant in NREM and at the supine position during sleep. FC, *BPM* heart rate in beat per minute; *AC* central apnea; *AO* obstructive apnea; *AM* mixed apnea; *HIPO* hypopnea; Estagio: sleep stage; *Pos* positioning; *MIC* microfone; *Mov Per* leg movement; *despertar* arousal. Body position—*S* supine, *E* left lateral decubitus. (Source: author's collection)

After the second polysomnography (performed without mandibular advancement device), and because of complaints of sleep interruptions and diurnal drowsiness, the patient was referred for PAP therapy.

9.2 Therapeutic Intervention

The patient started pressure therapy using automatic CPAP (5.4–8.0 cmH_2O) with a medium size AirFit P10 ResMed nose mask. Despite satisfactory treatment results, the patient complained of excessive leakage of air from the mouth (Table 9.1).

It was suggested that the adhesive tape method (Fig. 9.3) be used temporarily to stimulate the orbicularis oris muscle to hold a lip seal while sleeping. The patient was also referred for myofunctional therapy, considering that the change in the muscle tone of the upper airway muscles may be the causal factor for mouth opening when using CPAP [1].

Table 9.1 Presents the main results of the various approaches to the use of CPAP (nasal mask, nasal mask with oral tape, and oronasal mask). CPAP pressure has been adjusted to offer treatment benefits and patient comfort. We can observe the residual AHI control in all approaches. OSA severity is defined as mild for apnea-hypopnea index (AHI) ≥ 5 and < 15, moderate for AHI ≥ 15 and ≤ 30, and severe for AHI > 30/h. [2, 3] Source: Author's collection

	27 days-period of CPAP use	32 days-period of CPAP use	11 days-period of CPAP use
Usage days/total days (percentile of more than 4 h of usage per night)	26/27 (88%)	32/32 (96%)	11/11 (63%)
Mask	Nasal	Nasal with mouth tape	Oronasal
Pressure – cmH_2O	5.4–8.0	5.4–7.4	5.4–8.2
Median pressure – cmH_2O	7.1	6.7	7.6
Pressure 95th percentile – cmH_2O	7.9	7.3	8.2
Average usage (total days) – Hours	6:08	6:18	5:24
Median usage (days used) - hours	6:40	6:25	5:52
Expiratory relief	Off	Off	Off
95th percentile leaks – L/min	27.6	24.0	0.0
Median leaks – L/min	9.0	6.0	0.0
Events per hour (residual AHI)	0.9	1.1	3.3
Central apnea index	0.4	0.5	0.6
Obstructive apnea index	0.0	0.0	1.1
Obstructive hypopnea index	0.3	0.5	0.8
Unknown apnea index	0.0	0.0	0.0

Fig. 9.3 A method of closing the mouth with a skin-friendly tape to encourage lip tightness and control mouth leakage during the use of CPAP, used by the patient. (Source: own work)

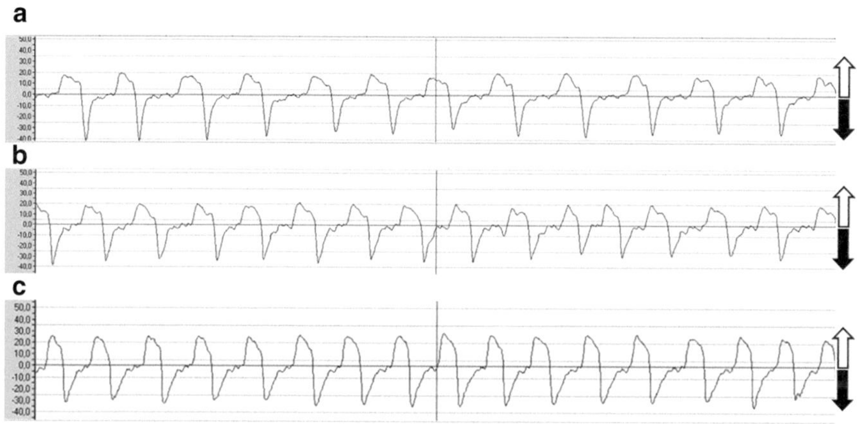

Fig. 9.4 Provide examples of the respiratory flow curve using a nasal mask without the mouth tape (**a**), a nasal mask with mouth tape (**b**), and an oronasal mask (**c**). The 95th percentile leak was 27.6, 24.0, and 0.0 at A, B, and C respectively. The more leak control, the less "spiculated" pattern presents the expiratory flow curve (black arrow) and the wider is the inspiratory flow curve (white arrow). Source: Author's collection

The patient obtained improved oral air leakage control when using the CPAP with the mouth tape (Table 9.1). Unfortunately, he started but failed to follow-up on functional myotherapy.

Despite not presenting complaints regarding the use of adhesive tape in conjunction with pressure therapy, the patient was invited to try the oronasal interface (AirFit F30i ResMed medium size), where he presented excellent control of air leakage. However, the patient reported discomfort with the oronasal mask and preferred to keep the adhesive tape together with the nasal mask when using CPAP. Table 9.1 shows the CPAP results with the different approaches used.

Interestingly, it was possible to observe in the respiratory flow curve during sleep how, with the air leakage control through the different methods used (nasal mask without the mouth tape, nasal mask with mouth tape, and an oronasal mask), the expiratory flow curve became less "spiculated" and the inspiratory flow curve began to show an increase in its amplitude (Fig. 9.4).

Despite the studies showing the benefit of using the chinstrap in controlling oral leakage, [4] the patient refused to use this accessory concomitantly with the nasal mask. In the end, the patient chose to keep the adhesive tape together with the nasal mask when using CPAP.

Take Away Message

1. Unintentional air leakage from the mouth may contribute to patient discomfort when using CPAP.
2. Some methods can help control air leakage from the mouth while using CPAP, such as the use of skin-safe tape on the mouth, chinstrap, myofunctional therapy, and the oronasal mask.

3. Oral leakage control methods depend not only on their efficacy, but also on the availability and comfort of the patient to use the method.
4. Assessing the breathing flow curve during sleep is an excellent practice for checking the results of oral leak control methods in a more objective manner.

References

1. Lebret M, Martinot JB, Arnol N, Zerillo D, Tamisier R, Pepin JL, et al. Factors contributing to unintentional leak during CPAP treatment: a systematic review. Chest. 2017;151(3):707–19. https://doi.org/10.1016/j.chest.2016.11.049.
2. Berry RBBR, Gamaldo CE, Harding SM, Marcus CL, Vaughn BV, Tangredi MM, for the American Academy of Sleep Medicine. The AASM manual for the scoring of sleep and associated events: rules, terminology and technical specifications. Darien, IL: www.aasmnet.org; 2012.
3. Berry RB, Brooks R, Gamaldo C, Harding SM, Lloyd RM, Quan SF, et al. AASM scoring manual updates for 2017 (version 2.4). J Clin Sleep Med. 2017;13(5):665–6. https://doi.org/10.5664/jcsm.6576.
4. Bachour A, Hurmerinta K, Maasilta P. Mouth closing device (chinstrap) reduces mouth leak during nasal CPAP. Sleep Med. 2004;5(3):261–7. https://doi.org/10.1016/j.sleep.2003.11.004.

Chapter 10
Case Report: Obstructive Sleep Apnea and Obesity Hypoventilation Syndrome

10.1 Patient Information

A 26-year-old woman, BMI 58.1 kg/m^2, complained of morning fatigue, snoring, and reported worsening of her breathing over the past 2 months. She explains that dyspnea sometimes occurs during sleep and is associated with nightmares. The patient also had a medical record of epilepsy and obsessive-compulsive behavior disorder. Aripiprazole, sertraline, and alprazolam are utilized daily.

She underwent video-EEG monitoring (traditional 10–20 electrode placement system). Background activity during wakefulness revealed a posterior rhythm of 9–10 Hz. During the assessment, no clinical and/or electrographic seizures occurred. The evaluation found a slight disorganization of basal activity in the anterior and middle temporal region to the right. Epileptiform paroxysms of sharp waves, of moderate to high amplitude, were also noted amidst irregular slow waves of projection in the right temporal region, with maximum electronegativity oscillating mainly between the zygomatic (Zig2) and anterior temporal (FT8) electrodes, activated by drowsiness and sleep.

The patient was also referred for diagnostic polysomnography that showed a marked increase in the apnea/hypopnea index (92.6/h) with the occurrence of central apneas (8.0), mixed apneas (4.0), obstructive apneas (24.0), and a predominance of hypopneas (406 hypopnea events, and a hypopnea index of 85.0/h). Basal oxygen saturation was 92%. Average oxygen saturation overnight was 87%, minimum SaO_2 was 60%, and 69.9% of the total sleep time remained with saturation below 90%, The patient presented an increased number of awakenings (91.9/h), latency for the N2 sleep stage was about 22.5 min and REM sleep latency was about 97.5 min. The sleep efficiency was 82.6%. Sleep architecture presented N1: 0.7%; N2: 79.2%; N3: 6.3%; REM: 13.6%. The examination was carried out in ambient air to better evaluate respiratory events.

V. S. Piccin, *Monitoring Positive Pressure Therapy in Sleep-Related Breathing Disorders*, https://doi.org/10.1007/978-3-031-50292-7_10

The sleep test was compatible with severe sleep apnea. Likewise, the patient's sleep test and clinical condition indicated the possibility of obesity hypoventilation concomitant with sleep-disordered breathing. Following evaluation of the polysomnography test results, the patient was referred to positive airway pressure (PAP) therapy.

10.2 Therapeutic Intervention

The patient underwent a PAP test using a CPAP device coupled to an oximetry module, several nights, with a fixed CPAP pressure beginning at 8.0 cmH_2O. She was wearing a pillow mask AirFit P10 ResMed, small size. The patient underwent 7-day CPAP monitoring with OSA resolution and excellent compliance results (Table 10.1). It is very important to note that all therapy adjustments were done remotely. Currently, the remote monitoring system, for patients who use sleep pressure therapy, is an essential tool for rapid verification of PAP and therapeutic adjustment. This system even allows the visualization of oximetry data throughout the night when the oximetry module is coupled to the positive pressure device [1, 2]. In addition to data monitoring through the telemonitoring system, the patient was asked daily, by telephone contact, about her comfort with the pressure therapy the night before, and the pressure parameters were only adjusted based on the patient's comfort report and with patient consent.

At 14.0 cmH_2O, the resolution of apneic events (which had already occurred with a therapeutic pressure of 8.6 cmH_2O) and improved hypoventilation could be

Table 10.1 Nights when PAP treatment was tested, with different CPAP pressure parameters during sleep

	Night 1	Night 2	Night 3	Night 4	Night 5	Night 6	Night 7
CPAP pressure	*8.0 cmH_2O*	*8.6 cmH_2O*	*9.6 cmH_2O*	*11.0 cmH_2O*	*12.0 cmH_2O*	*13.0 cmH_2O*	*14.0 cmH_2O*
SaO_2 minimum	*85*	*87*	*85*	*68*	*72*	*81*	*84*
SaO_2 median	*92*	*93*	*92*	*93*	*93*	*93*	*93*
SaO_2 maximum	*98*	*98*	*96*	*98*	*100*	*98*	*97*
Time $SaO_2 < 90\%$ (hours)	*00:17*	*00:20*	*00:40*	*00:24*	*00:15*	*00:32*	*00:04*
AHI	*6.5*	*0.0*	*0.1*	*0.9*	*0.2*	*0.0*	*0.2*
CPAP usage (hours)	*05:59*	*07:26*	*07:18*	*08:07*	*06:42*	*06:36*	*06:58*
Leak (l/min at 95 percentile)	*9.6*	*1.2*	*2.4*	*2.4*	*3.6*	*3.6*	*4.8*
ODI	*9*	*4*	*6*	*4*	*5*	*2*	*2*

PAP positive airway pressure, *CPAP* continuous positive airway pressure, *SaO_2* oxygen saturation of arterial blood, *AHI* apnea-hypopnea index, *ODI* oxygen desaturation index verified. The pressure strategy adopted followed the recommendations of the American Thoracic Society (ATS), where studies have observed that ambulatory stable patients with obesity hypoventilation and high apnea-hypopnea index may be adequately responsive to CPAP (Fig. 10.1) [3, 4].

After the CPAP test, a test was also performed using the pressure device in bilevel therapeutic mode (IPAP 15.0 cmH_2O and EPAP 8.0 cmH_2O); however, the patient reported discomfort and was very resistant to proceed with the tests in that pressure mode, with a clear preference for using the CPAP device.

It was interesting to observe that at a CPAP of 14 cmH_2O, even with a respiratory disturbance, oxygen desaturation does not occur, according to the reading of the oximetry module attached to the device (Fig. 10.2). This finding is in line with the ATS guideline, which favors the use of CPAP over NIV for approximately two-thirds of patients with severe OSA concomitant with hypoventilation due to obesity. According to that guideline, although noninvasive ventilation monitoring (i.e., transcutaneous CO_2) theoretically should be added to SaO_2 monitoring for PAP titration or adjustment, no comparative studies were found using SaO_2 monitoring with or without non-invasive CO_2 monitoring. This domain needs further investigation. And often healthcare professionals need to consider options based on resource availability [3].

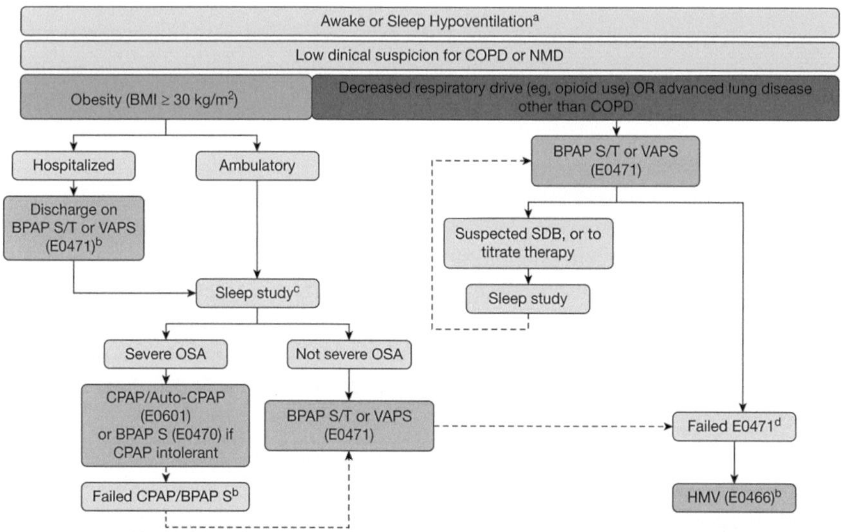

[a] **Awake hypoventilation** defined by $Paco_2 \geq 45$ mm Hg or equivalent method of diagnosis, OR **Sleep hypoventilation** defined by ≥ 10 mm Hg increase from baseline awake Pco_2, AND to a value ≥ 50 mm Hg for ≥ 10 min, OR $Pco_2 \geq 55$ mm Hg for ≥ 10 min. (Alternative methods for diagnosing hypoventilation may be based on venous blood gas, end-tidal co_2, or transcutaneous $co_2 \geq 50$ mm Hg.).
[b] In certain circumstances, patients may need to be discharged from the hospital on VAPS-AE or HMV or may require HMV without having failed BPAP S/T or VAPS (see text for summary of new suggestions).
[c] For ongoing coverage of E0471 following hospital discharge, a reassessment with a provider within 3 months is required and a sleep study should be performed to assess appropriateness of PAP modality.
[d] Therapy failure defined as persistent hypercapnia or symptoms following 3 months of adequate adherence to prescribed PAP therapy.

Fig. 10.1 Provides a flow diagram for suggested indications for outpatient NIV support for awake or sleep hypoventilation. (Source: Mokhlesi B et al., 2021 (with permission) [4])

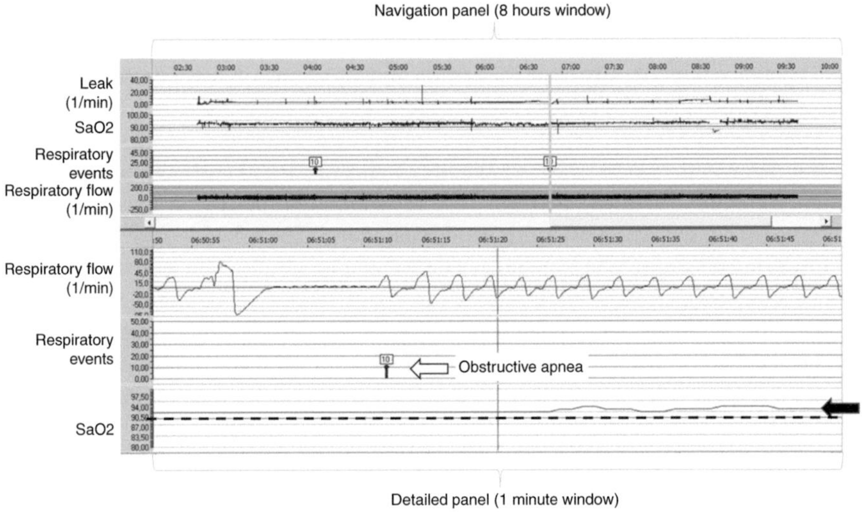

Fig. 10.2 In this figure, we can see that, at a CPAP of 14 cmH$_2$O, even with a respiratory disturbance, oxygen desaturation does not occur, according to the reading of the oximetry module attached to the device. Saturation remains higher than 90% after obstructive apnea (dotted line). (Source: author's collection)

At follow-up, the patient continued with excellent CPAP compliance, reporting significant improvement in mood and daytime sleepiness with the use of positive airway therapy.

Take Away Message

1. Evidence-based practice is critical for effective clinical management.
2. Currently, positive pressure devices provide technologies that enable remote monitoring and treatment adaptations quickly and accurately.
3. The oximetry module associated with positive pressure device is an essential resource for the proper monitoring of patients in the sleep field. The statistical report indicating the resolution of respiratory events throughout the night does not indicate improvement in ventilatory disorders, and health professionals should be aware of this.
4. The evaluation of the flow curve throughout the night, associated with the oximetry signal, is a powerful tool that allows assessing whether any desaturations are occurring due to sleep apneas or not.

References

1. Schutte-Rodin S. Telehealth, telemedicine, and obstructive sleep apnea. Sleep Med Clin. 2020;15(3):359–75. https://doi.org/10.1016/j.jsmc.2020.05.003.

2. Weaver TE. Novel aspects of CPAP treatment and interventions to improve CPAP adherence. J Clin Med. 2019;8(12):2220. https://doi.org/10.3390/jcm8122220.
3. Mokhlesi B, Masa JF, Brozek JL, Gurubhagavatula I, Murphy PB, Piper AJ, et al. Evaluation and management of obesity hypoventilation syndrome. An official American Thoracic Society clinical practice guideline. Am J Respir Crit Care Med. 2019;200(3):e6–e24. https://doi.org/10.1164/rccm.201905-1071ST.
4. Mokhlesi B, Won CH, Make BJ, Selim BJ, Sunwoo BY, OTE P. Optimal noninvasive medicare access promotion: patients with hypoventilation syndromes a technical expert panel report from the American College of Chest Physicians, the American Association for Respiratory Care, the American Academy of sleep medicine, and the American Thoracic Society. Chest. 2021;160:e377. https://doi.org/10.1016/j.chest.2021.06.083.

Index

V. S. Piccin, *Monitoring Positive Pressure Therapy in Sleep-Related Breathing Disorders*, https://doi.org/10.1007/978-3-031-50292-7

MIX
Papier aus verantwortungsvollen Quellen
Paper from responsible sources
FSC® C105338

If you have any concerns about our products,
you can contact us on
ProductSafety@springernature.com

In case Publisher is established outside the EU,
the EU authorized representative is:
Springer Nature Customer Service Center GmbH
Europaplatz 3, 69115 Heidelberg, Germany

Printed by Libri Plureos GmbH
in Hamburg, Germany